The Pocket Atlas of Trigger Points

The Pocket Atlas of Trigger Points

A User-Friendly Guide to Muscle Anatomy, Pain Patterns, and the Myofascial Network for Students, Practitioners, and Patients

Simeon Niel-Asher

lotus
publishing

Chichester, England

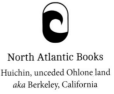

North Atlantic Books
Huichin, unceded Ohlone land
aka Berkeley, California

First published in 2023 by
Lotus Publishing
Apple Tree Cottage, Inlands Road, Nutbourne, Chichester, PO18 8RJ, and
North Atlantic Books
Huichin, unceded Ohlone land
aka Berkeley, California

Illustrations Amanda Williams
Text Design Medlar Publishing Solutions Pvt Ltd., India
Cover Design Chris Fulcher
Printed and Bound in India by Replika Press Pvt Ltd.

The Pocket Atlas of Trigger Points: A User-Friendly Guide to Muscle Anatomy, Pain Patterns, and the Myofascial Network for Students, Practitioners, and Patients is sponsored and published by North Atlantic Books, an educational nonprofit based on the unceded Ohlone land Huichin (*aka* Berkeley, CA), that collaborates with partners to develop cross-cultural perspectives, nurture holistic views of art, science, the humanities, and healing, and seed personal and global transformation by publishing work on the relationship of body, spirit, and nature.

North Atlantic Books' publications are distributed to the US trade and internationally by Penguin Random House Publishers Services. For further information, visit our website at www.northatlanticbooks.com.

MEDICAL DISCLAIMER: The following information is intended for general information purposes only. Individuals should always see their health care provider before administering any suggestions made in this book. Any application of the material set forth in the following pages is at the reader's discretion and is their sole responsibility.

British Library Cataloging-in-Publication Data
A CIP record for this book is available from the British Library
ISBN 978 1 913088 12 5 (Lotus Publishing)
ISBN 978 1 62317 934 2 (North Atlantic Books)
ISBN 978 1 62317 935 9 (Ebook)

Library of Congress Cataloging-in-Publication Data
Names: Niel-Asher, Simeon, author.
Title: The pocket atlas of trigger points : a user-friendly guide to muscle
   anatomy, pain patterns, and the myofascial network for students,
   practitioners, and patients / Simeon Niel-Asher.
Description: Chichester, England : Lotus Publishing ; Berkeley, California :
   North Atlantic Books, 2023. | Includes bibliographical references.
Identifiers: LCCN 2022059896 (print) | LCCN 2022059897 (ebook) |
   ISBN 9781913088125 (Lotus Publishing) | ISBN 9781623179342
   (North Atlantic Books) | ISBN 9781623179359 (ebook)
Subjects: MESH: Trigger Points | Muscles--physiology | Myofascial Pain
   Syndromes--therapy | Handbook
Classification: LCC QP321 (print) | LCC QP321 (ebook) | NLM WE 39 |
   DDC 612.7/4--dc23/eng/20230119
LC record available at https://lccn.loc.gov/2022059896
LC ebook record available at https://lccn.loc.gov/2022059897

Contents

Introduction   7

**Chapter 1—Trigger Points and
Trigger Point Formation   13**
  Nutritional and
    Biochemical Factors   15
  Muscle Morphology
    and Trigger Points   16
  Trigger Point Symptoms   18
  Trigger Point Classification 19
  Trigger Point Formation
    and Posture   21
  Trigger Points, Fascia,
    and Myofascial Meridians   24
  Plotting the Pain   26
  Schematic Interpretation
    of Pain Maps and Muscles
    Affected   28

**Chapter 2—Muscles of the
Face, Head, and Neck   37**
  Occipitofrontalis   38
  Orbicularis Oculi   40
  Corrugator Supercilii   42
  Procerus   43
  Buccinator   44
  Zygomaticus Major   45
  Masseter   46
  Temporalis   48
  Lateral Pterygoid   50
  Medial Pterygoid   51
  Platysma   53
  Digastric   54
  Omohyoid   56
  Longus Colli   57
  Longus Capitis   59
  Scalenes   60

  Sternocleidomastoid   62
  Suboccipital Group   65
  Trigger Points and
    Headaches   67

**Chapter 3—Muscles of the
Trunk and Spine   69**
  Erector Spinae
    (Sacrospinalis)   70
  Posterior Cervical Muscles   72
  Multifidus and Rotatores   74
  Splenius Capitis and
    Splenius Cervicis   76
  Intercostals   78
  Serratus Posterior
    Superior   80
  Serratus Posterior
    Inferior   81
  Diaphragm   83
  External Oblique   84
  Transversus Abdominis   86
  Rectus Abdominis   88
  Quadratus Lumborum   90
  Iliopsoas   92
  Pelvic Floor Muscles   94
  Trigger Points and
    Low Back Pain   95

**Chapter 4—Muscles of the
Shoulder and Arm   97**
  Trapezius   98
  Levator Scapulae   100
  Rhomboids   101
  Serratus Anterior   103
  Pectoralis Minor   105
  Subclavius   106
  Pectoralis Major   108
  Sternalis   110

Latissimus Dorsi 111
Deltoid 113
Supraspinatus 115
Infraspinatus 117
Teres Minor 118
Subscapularis 120
Teres Major 121
Biceps Brachii 123
Brachialis 125
Coracobrachialis 127
Triceps Brachii 128
Anconeus 130
Trigger Points and Frozen
Shoulder Syndrome
(Adhesive Capsulitis) 131

**Chapter 5—Muscles of the
Forearm and Hand** **133**
Pronator Teres 134
Palmaris Longus 135
Wrist Flexors 136
Pronator Quadratus 138
Brachioradialis 139
Wrist Extensors 140
Extensor Digitorum 142
Supinator 144
Abductor Pollicis Longus 146
Extensor Indicis 147
Opponens Pollicis and
Adductor Pollicis 148
Abductor Pollicis Brevis 150
Small Hand Muscles 151
Trigger Points and
Carpal Tunnel Syndrome 155

**Chapter 6—Muscles of the
Hip and Thigh** **157**
Gluteus Maximus 158
Tensor Fasciae Latae 160
Gluteus Medius 161
Gluteus Minimus 163
Piriformis 164
"GIGO" Muscles 166

Gemelli 167
Obturator Internus 168
Quadratus Femoris 169
Sartorius 170
Quadriceps 172
Gracilis 175
Pectineus 176
Obturator Externus 177
Adductors 178
Hamstrings 180
Trigger Points and
Osteoarthritis of the Hip 183
Trigger Points and
Buckling Knee 184

**Chapter 7—Muscles of the
Leg and Foot** **185**
Tibialis Anterior 186
Extensor Digitorum
Longus and Extensor
Hallucis Longus 187
Fibulares 189
Gastrocnemius 191
Plantaris 192
Soleus 194
Popliteus 195
Flexor Digitorum
Longus and Flexor
Hallucis Longus 197
Tibialis Posterior 199
Superficial Muscles
of the Foot 200
Deep Muscles of the Foot 203
Trigger Points and
Heel Pain 206

*Appendix I: Dermatomes and
Sensory Nerve Supply* 207
*Appendix II: Super Trigger
Points* 213
References 215

Introduction

This pocket atlas is designed in quick reference format to offer useful information about the muscle anatomy and referred pain patterns of the trigger points relating to the main skeletal muscles, which are central to massage, bodywork, and physical therapy.

The book is also practical for patients who wish to work with their practitioner and help them understand their underlying trigger points. At the end of Chapters 2 to 7, I examine conditions that commonly occur in the general population.

X Marks the Spot

While I have included the location of the most common trigger points, please note that these are not exact. A number of factors influence the location. Fascia—the connective tissue that binds us—is a continuum, and minor variations, for example, anatomy, posture, and weight bearing, will have an impact on the location and formation of trigger points.

The grapefruit principle: fascia holds everything in shape

All of our internal organs are literally surrounded by fascia. It permeates our entire bodies, in various surface layers as well as in the deeper layers. A colleague of mine, Thomas Myers, uses 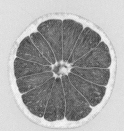 this vivid image of a grapefruit to illustrate the way that fascia holds the entire body in shape. The pulp of the grapefruit is enclosed in small detachments of white skin, and on the outside it is again surrounded by a solid white skin that fits snugly to the peel.

> If you were to remove all the pulp and leave only the white skin, you could reconstruct the entire fruit and its shape on the basis of this structure alone. The same principle applies to fascia and its function in the human body. It is possible to see how a person looks based solely on the connective tissue, without the flesh and bones. The same does not apply, however, to the skeleton.
>
> —R. Schleip, *Fascial Fitness*, Second Edition (2021).

In the "real world," you may well find that the trigger point location varies slightly from the dots on the muscles in Chapters 2 to 7. Varying the direction, amplitude, applicator forces, and even the patient position, will also have an impact on locating the trigger point.

There are a series of headings relating to each muscle/s, that are explained below.

Attachments
A muscle is usually attached to two bones that form a joint, and when the muscle contracts, it pulls the movable bone toward the stationary bone. All muscles have at least two attachments. The origin (red) and insertion (blue) of, for example, trapezius is shown in Figure 1.

Origin
The attachment that remains relatively immobile during muscular contraction. This is usually the end of the muscle which is fixed to the bone, thereby acting as an anchor for the muscle to pull its opposite end (insertion) toward this stable attachment.

Insertion
The attachment that moves, hence the opposite end of the muscle to the origin. For certain movements, when the insertion remains relatively fixed and the origin moves, the muscle is said to be performing a reversed action from

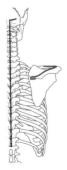

Figure 1: Origin and insertion of trapezius.

the origin to insertion. Generally, the origin is more proximal (toward the center of the body) and the insertion is more distal (toward the periphery of the body).

Nerve
This relates to the nerve that activates the muscle. There are subtle variations between texts regarding the nerve supply of individual muscles, but the suggestions in this book are compiled using a wide range of resources to produce a common reference point.

Action
The movement or effect caused when the muscle contracts.

Basic Functional Movement
Everyday activities to which the muscle contributes.

Referred Pain Patterns
Radiating zones of pain related to specific trigger points (Figure 2). Over 55% of commonly found trigger points are not located within their area of referred pain (DeLaune 2011).

Indications
Presenting symptoms, areas of dysfunction, or pain felt by the patient.

Causes
Exploring factors that may induce trigger point formation, such as postural patterns relating to work/sleep or habitual activities.

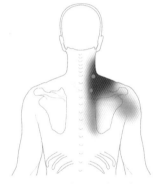

Figure 2: Referred pain patterns of levator scapulae.

Differential Diagnosis
Other conditions or dysfunctions are suggested as possible causes of the pain that may present similar signs and symptoms

Connections
Other muscle trigger points with similar patterns.

Stretching and Strengthening

Travell and Simons (1999) found that *active* trigger points benefited from stretching, but were usually aggravated by strengthening exercises, so work with your chosen practitioner and begin your treatment with stretching exercises.

Stretch

Stretching means that you are gently lengthening or "opening out" the muscle fibers, and has a host of benefits, including improved range of movement, increased power, diminished post-treatment soreness, and reduced fatigue. Usually two weeks of stretching for trigger point self-help will be sufficient before adding the strengthening exercises. Ideally you will be working with your health practitioner/physical therapist to work out the best protocol for you.

Stretching Guidelines

Stretching is a simple and effective activity. Slowly get into the stretch position and then hold each stretch for a minimum of 20 seconds, and then adhere to the following rules:

- Never stretch an injury or damaged soft tissue
- Do not bounce on a stretch
- Warm-up prior to stretching
- Stretch gently and slowly
- Stretch only to the point of tension
- Breathe slowly and easily

Strengthen (or Condition)

As mentioned, normally two weeks of stretching will be sufficient before adding strengthening exercises, but if your trigger points remain irritable, or you have night pain, wait until your symptoms have improved.

Strengthening (conditioning) the muscles improves their tolerance and stamina to exercise, helping to relieve pain, improve the function of the muscles, and prevent further injury. As a rule, strengthening a muscle occurs when you hold maximal muscle contraction for between five and ten seconds.

Self-Help Tools

A variety of self-help tools have been developed for manipulating trigger points (Figure 3). Each of these tools has a different effect—in general, they are designed either to apply pressure to a specific trigger point or to stretch out the muscles after treatment—and can be used while standing, sitting, lying, or side lying.

It is easy to overstimulate an active trigger point, so pressure should be applied slowly and gently until it is "just right." Hold the point until it softens or the pain subsides, and use your chosen tool(s) up to six times a day, depending on how chronic the problem is.

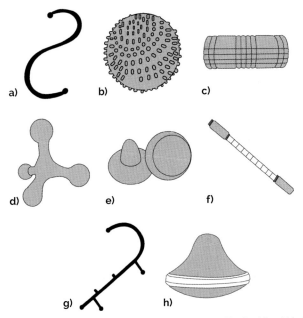

Figure 3: Self-help tools for manipulating trigger points, a) backnobber, b) ball, c) foam roller, d) four, e) knobble, f) one, g) theracane, h) tola.

CHAPTER 1

Trigger Points and Trigger Point Formation

Drs. Janet Travell and David Simons (1992) described a trigger point as "A highly irritable localized spot of exquisite tenderness in a nodule in a palpable taut band of (skeletal) muscle."

These hyperirritable localized spots can vary in size, and have been described as "tiny lumps," "little peas," and "large lumps"; they can be felt beneath the surface, embedded within the muscle fibers. If these spots are tender to pressure they may well be trigger points. The size of a trigger point nodule varies according to the size, shape, and type of muscle in which it is generated. What is consistent is that they are tender to pressure—so tender that when they are pressed, the patient often winces from the pain. This has been called the *jump sign*.

Myofascial trigger points may well be implicated in all types of musculoskeletal and mechanical muscular pain. Their presence has even been demonstrated in children and babies. Pain or symptoms may be directly due to active trigger points, or pain may "build up" over time from latent or inactive trigger points. Studies and investigations in selected patient populations have been carried out on various regions of the body. There is a growing amount of research evidence directly linking musculoskeletal pain to trigger points. A high prevalence of trigger points has been confirmed to be directly associated with myofascial pain, somatic dysfunction, psychological disturbance, and associated restricted daily functioning.

Etiology
Several possible trigger point mechanisms have been put forward (Dommerholt et al. 2006):

- Low-level muscle contractions
- Uneven intramuscular pressure distribution
- Direct trauma
- Unaccustomed eccentric contractions
- Eccentric contractions in unconditioned muscle
- Maximal or submaximal concentric contractions

Trigger points develop in the myofascia (hence the descriptor *myofascial trigger points* or MTPs), mainly in the center of the muscle belly where the motor end plate enters (primary or central). However, secondary or satellite trigger points often develop in a response to the primary trigger point. These satellite points often develop along fascial lines of stress, which may well be "built-in" at the time of embryogenesis.

External factors—such as aging, body morphology, posture, weight gain, or congenital malformation—also play a crucial role in trigger point manifestation and genesis.

Referred Radicular Pain and Trigger Point Maps

Much like pain from a damaged nerve, trigger point stimulation causes referred pain. There are, however, several key differences (Table 1.1). It is advisable to perform neurological testing to eliminate any neural involvement.

Table 1.1: Differences between neural and trigger point referred pain.

Neural (Radicular) Referred Pain	Trigger Point Referred Pain
Specific dermatomal pattern	Map may extend across several dermatomes
Loss of sensitivity in dermatome	No loss of sensitivity
Loss of motor power to the point of paralysis	Weakness but no power loss on testing
Not induced by local muscle tissue pressure	Induced with local muscle tissue pressure
Loss of deep tendon reflex	No loss of deep tendon reflex

Trigger point referred pain is different to the referred shoulder pain of appendicitis or a jaw/arm pain with a heart attack. When you hold a trigger point for 5–6 seconds, part or all of the map should activate.

Nutritional and Biochemical Factors

Simons et al. (1998) suggested that changes in biochemical inputs might influence trigger point formation and/or perpetuation (Table 1.2). Gerwin et al. (2004) expanded upon this, asserting that nutritional and biochemical factors may well both precipitate and maintain chronic myofascial pain and "must be" considered during treatment.

Table 1.2: Biomechanical factors. After Simons et al. (1998) and Gerwin (2004).

Factor	Influence
Allergic/hypersensitivity	May have a potentizing effect (Brostoff 1992).
Hormonal	Estrogen and thyroid deficiency may impact the endoplasmic environment, leading to increased trigger point development and/or perpetuation (Lowe & Honeyman-Lowe 1998).
Chronic viral, yeast and/or parasite infection	May increase the likelihood of trigger point formation (Ferguson & Gerwin 2004).
Vitamin C deficiency	May perpetuate trigger point longevity.
Iron deficiency (ferritin)	10–15% of people with chronic myofascial pain syndromes may be iron deficient (Simons et al. 1999). Serum levels of 15–20 ng/ml indicate depletion, but even levels below 50 ng/ml may be significant (Gerwin et al. 2004).
Vitamin B1, B6, B12 deficiency	May increase tiredness, fatigue, and chronic trigger point formation.
Magnesium and zinc deficiency	Levels in the lower realm of normal may be low for some people.
Vitamin D deficiency	Implicated in almost 90% of patients with chronic musculoskeletal pain (Plotnikoff 2003).
Cytochrome oxidase	Lowered levels are common in patients with myalgia. Associated with tiredness, coldness, extreme fatigue with exercise, and muscle pain.
Folic acid	May sufficiently change the internal endoplasmic environment to increase trigger point development and/or perpetuation.

Muscle Morphology and Trigger Points

Trigger points tend to develop in the belly of the muscle around the neuromuscular junctions (NMJs) or motor end plates (MEPs), Figure 1.1.

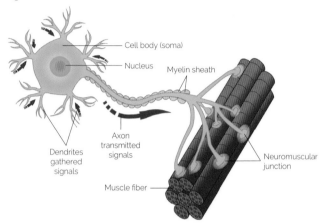

Figure 1.1: Motor unit of a skeletal muscle.

Muscles come in a variety of shapes according to the arrangement of their fascicles. The reason for this variation is to provide optimum mechanical efficiency for a muscle in relation to its position and action.

The most common arrangement of fascicles yields muscle shapes which can be described as parallel, pennate, convergent, and circular, with each of these shapes having further sub-categories. Trigger points may occur simultaneously in multiple heads of a bipennate or multipennate muscle (Figure 1.2).

Trigger Points and Muscle Fiber Type

All muscles contain a blend of type 1 and type 2 fibers (Janda 2005; Lewit 1999). This has a direct correlation with how chronic symptoms might develop if left untreated.

1. Type 1 fibers are postural and tend to respond to stress or overuse by shortening and becoming hypertonic. A trigger point in a

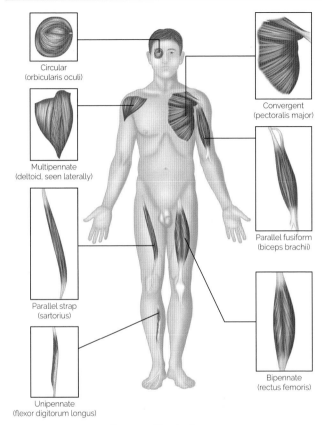

Circular
(orbicularis oculi)

Convergent
(pectoralis major)

Multipennate
(deltoid, seen laterally)

Parallel fusiform
(biceps brachii)

Parallel strap
(sartorius)

Unipennate
(flexor digitorum longus)

Bipennate
(rectus femoris)

Figure 1.2: Muscle shapes.

muscle with a high percentage of type 1 fibers may take longer to respond to treatment.

2. Type 2 fibers are built for explosive, short-term activity and tend to become weak, atrophic, and hypertonic under chronic or sustained endurance. A trigger point in a muscle with a high percentage of type 2 fibers may respond more rapidly to treatment.

Trigger Point Symptoms

Referred Pain Patterns

Pain is a complex symptom experienced differently and individually. However, *referred* pain is the defining symptom of a myofascial trigger point.

Referred pain from a myofascial trigger point is a distinct and discrete pattern or map of pain. This map is consistent, and has no racial or gender differences, because stimulating an active trigger point generates the pain.

Patients describe referred pain in this map as having a "deep" and "aching" quality; movement may sometimes exacerbate symptoms, making the pain "sharper." An example of this might be a headache. The patient often describes a pattern of pain, or ache, which can sometimes be aggravated and made sharper by moving the head and neck. The intensity of pain will vary according to the following factors (this list is not exhaustive):

- Location (attachment points are more sensitive)
- Degree of trigger point irritability
- Active or latent trigger points
- Primary or satellite trigger points
- Site of trigger point (some areas are more sensitive)
- Associated tissue damage
- Location/host tissue stiffness or flexibility
- Aging
- Chronicity of trigger point

Maintaining Factors

The presence of one or several of the following factors may well present some difficulty in eliminating trigger points over the long term:

- Aging
- Posture (including work)
- Obesity
- Anorexia
- Scar tissue (post-surgical)
- Sports, hobbies, habits
- Stress and strain patterns
- Metabolic disorders
- Disease or illness

- Sleep disturbance (including apnea)
- Iron deficiency
- Vitamin and mineral deficiency (folic acid, C, D, B1, B6, B12, iron, magnesium, and zinc)
- Congenital (bony) anomaly
- Type of muscle fiber
- Direction/orientation of muscle fiber
- Muscle shape/morphology (fusiform, etc.)
- Psychological factors—depression, anxiety, anger, and feelings of hopelessness
- Chronicity of trigger point

Trigger Point Classification

The current thinking is that trigger points are considered to be either *inactive* (or latent) or *active*. However, in the older literature they are also described according to location, tenderness, and chronicity as *central* (or *primary*), *satellite* (or *secondary*), *attachment*, and *diffuse*.

Inactive (or Latent) Trigger Points

This applies to lumps and nodules that feel like trigger points. These can develop anywhere in the body and are often secondary. However, these trigger points are not painful, and do not elicit a referred pain pathway. The presence of inactive trigger points within muscles may lead to increased "muscular stiffness." It has been suggested that these points are more common in those who live a sedentary lifestyle (Starlanyl & Copeland 2001). It is worth noting that these points may reactivate if the central or primary trigger point is (re)stimulated; reactivation may also occur following trauma and injury.

Active Trigger Points

This can apply to central and satellite trigger points. A variety of stimulants, such as forcing muscular activity through pain, can activate an inactive trigger point. This situation is common when activity is increased after a road traffic accident (RTA), where multiple and diffuse trigger points may have developed. The term denotes that the trigger point is both tender to palpation and elicits a referred pain pattern.

Central (or Primary) Trigger Points

These are the most well-established and "florid" points when they are *active*, and are usually what people refer to when they talk about trigger points. Central trigger points always exist in the center of the muscle belly, where the motor end plate enters the muscle.

Note: Muscle shape and fiber arrangement is of importance in this regard, e.g., there may be *several* central points in multipennate muscles. Also, if muscle fibers run diagonally, this may lead to variations in trigger point location.

Satellite (or Secondary) Trigger Points
Trigger points may be "created" as a response to the central trigger point in neighboring muscles that lie within the *referred pain zone*. In such cases, the primary trigger point is still the key to therapeutic intervention: the satellite trigger points often resolve once the primary point has been effectively rendered *inactive*. As a corollary, it is also true that satellite points may prove resilient to treatment until the primary *central* focus is weakened; this is often the case in the paraspinal and/or abdominal muscles.

Attachment Trigger Points
The area where the tendon inserts into the bone (tendo-osseous junction) is often "exquisitely" tender (Simons et al. 1998; Davies 2004). This may well be the result of the existing forces traveling across these regions. It has also been suggested by the same authors that this may result from an associated chronic, active myofascial trigger point. This is because the tenderness has been demonstrated to reduce once the primary central trigger point has been treated; in such cases, the point is described as an *attachment* trigger point.

Ligamentous Trigger Points
There is some evidence that ligaments may develop trigger points but the relationships are not clear. For example, the sacrotuberous and sacrospinous ligaments can refer pain down to the heel and the iliolumbar ligament can refer pain down to the groin and even into the testicles or vagina (Hacket 1991).

Diffuse Trigger Points
Trigger points can sometimes occur where multiple satellite trigger points exist secondary to multiple central trigger points. This is often the case when there is a severe postural deformity, such as a scoliosis, and an entire quadrant of the body is involved. In this scenario, the secondary points are said to be *diffuse*. These diffuse trigger points often develop along lines of altered *stress* and/or *strain* patterns.

Trigger Point Formation and Posture

Poor posture is a powerful "activator and perpetuator" of myofascial trigger points (Simons et al. 1998) and is always worth considering in chronic trigger point syndromes. Postural muscles tend to have a greater percentage of type 1 fibers; this characteristic may lead to a more resistant type of trigger point.

It is a fact that in the developed world many occupations involve prolonged sitting, often at a computer screen. For many people, long and monotonous days spent in front of a computer screen often lead to chronic and maladapted postures. Where possible, it is essential to identify the postural abnormalities (Figure 1.3) and how they impact the patient's symptoms, and offer to remedy the situation via ergonomic advice, treatment, and/or exercise.

The most common mechanical maladaptations are

- Head-forward posture and round shoulders
- Head to one side—telephone posture
- Occupational/ergonomic stressors
- Slouched standing and "sway-back" posture
- Slouched sitting (e.g., computer screen/ergonomics)
- Cross-legged sitting
- Habitual postures
- Driving position
- Scoliosis
- Joint hypermobility
- Lifting/carrying
- Primary short lower extremity (PSLE)

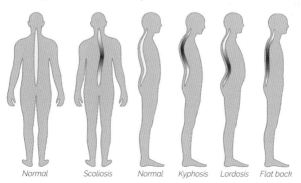

Normal *Scoliosis* *Normal* *Kyphosis* *Lordosis* *Flat back*

Figure 1.3: Typically seen pathological curvatures of the spine.

Posture as a Predisposing Factor

Poor posture has been implicated in a range of clinical complaints and it plays a crucial role in maintaining myofascial structural integrity and thus is directly connected to trigger point activity. Faulty sitting and/or standing postures are both a pathogenic and maintaining factor for trigger point activity. Advice and exercises for posture is often the key to unlocking both *central* and *satellite* points.

Sleeping Posture

We all frequently assume strange postures at night, which will sometimes be adopted to reduce the pain from either active or stiff latent trigger points (Figure 1.4). In such cases, patients often opt for a sleeping position that shortens the affected muscle: for example, they sleep with either the hands above the head (supraspinatus), or the

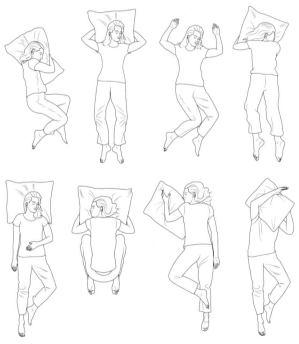

Figure 1.4: Sleeping postures likely to contribute toward trigger point formation.

arms folded over the chest (pectoralis major). In other cases, it may be that the sleeping position is a pathogenic or a maintaining factor.

Work Posture

Some patients may have manual or repetitive activities in the workplace, which may well have a role to play in trigger point pathogenesis or maintenance. Figure 1.5 illustrates an ideal sitting posture at work.

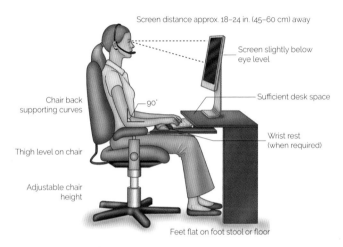

Figure 1.5: Ideal sitting posture at work.

Habitual Activity, Hobbies, and Sports

Similarly, it is important to ask the patient if they perform any repetitive or habitual activities apart from at work. Standing all day on one leg, for example, may well overload the tensor fasciae latae muscle. Sitting in a cross-legged position may affect a range of muscles, such as the hip flexors (iliopsoas), the buttock muscles (gluteals and piriformis), and the thigh muscles (quadriceps). Heavy smokers may develop trigger points in the shoulder (deltoid) and arm (biceps brachii) muscles.

Certain hobbies and sports may also lead to an increased incidence of trigger point pathogenesis. It is important to enquire carefully about such activities. What is their level of competence? Do they warm up, and cool down? How competitive are they? Is their level of activity realistic for their age? Posture? Body type? Physical health? You may want to explore these areas further. It is often useful to run through these activities and set the patient certain *activity goals* to achieve in between treatment sessions.

Trigger Points, Fascia, and Myofascial Meridians

> *The fascia is the place to look for the cause of disease and the place to consult and begin the action of remedies in all diseases.*
> —Dr. Andrew Taylor Still—founder
> of Osteopathic Medicine, Kirksville, Missouri

Identifying and treating myofascial trigger points can be uniquely effective therapeutically; trigger points, however, rarely develop in isolation and may return if the underlying cause is not identified and addressed. Long-standing trigger points may lead to secondary (and even tertiary) changes in the nervous system (sensitization) and to trigger point formation elsewhere remote from the original problem.

While trigger points may develop as a result of trauma, injury, or overuse, there may be other mechanisms at play.

Holding Patterns
Patients may come with acute or chronic symptoms, but, whatever the origin, the body's myofascial framework adapts and changes in a protective "holding pattern." Over time the "normal" muscle functioning fails, often resulting in multiple trigger point formation. The longer a problem persists, the more rigid these patterns may become. Chains of sarcomeres fail and chronic recalcitrant trigger points form. Peripheral and central sensitization play a role in maintaining this holding pattern, but so does the adapted myofascial infrastructure.

Context
It is important therefore to see trigger points in context: What is the body trying to achieve? Why has its tolerance/compensation broken down? Where and what is the central or core issue? I encourage my students to think like detectives: find the "tissues that are causing the symptoms" and then reflect and observe how the body has adapted over time to compensate. This requires a holistic view of the patient's body, organs, bones, and supporting tissues, as well as their posture, nutrition, occupation, psychological state, and general wellbeing.

Trigger Points Tend to Develop Along "Myofascial Meridians"

Clinically, trigger points (and super trigger points) tend to emerge in the myofascia along certain predetermined lines of force, or meridians. The reasons for this have been suggested by Thomas Myers (2001) and are based on the earlier work of Ida Rolf. The concept of "myofascial channels," or chains, helps to explain the way the body dissipates and distributes forces from right to left, up to down, and deep to superficial. It is useful therefore to understand and visualize these myofascial meridian train lines (Figure 1.6).

Muscles do not operate in isolation, but might be regarded as the contractile elements within a myofascial continuum, which runs throughout the body. These meridian maps may help to explain how and why the development of primary, central trigger points in one area of the body may lead to secondary or satellite trigger points distally.

To explore myofascial meridians further, refer to *Anatomy Trains: Myofascial Meridians for Manual Therapists and Movement Professionals* (Myers, T. 2020).

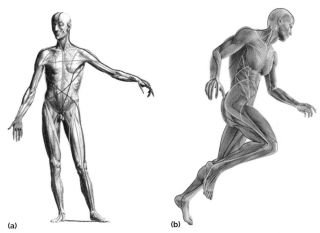

(a) (b)

Figure 1.6: The Anatomy Trains Myofascial Meridians. (a) The original Anatomy Trains map, drawn like the London Underground lines to show the pathways by which compensation can be shifted from one part of the body to another, quite distant part to affect the global postural pattern. (b) This more dynamic and recent rendering of the Anatomy Trains map encourages us to ask ourselves whether we are able to access, establish and make full use of the functional efficiencies afforded by these lines. Taken from *Fascial Release for Structural Balance, Revised Edition* (Myers, T., & Earls, J. 2017), courtesy of Anatomy Trains.

Plotting the Pain

Use these blank charts to plot your area of pain, and then compare them with the pain referral patterns given in Chapters 2 to 7. Note your pain intensity over a period of a few days or weeks and note any shift in pattern or level of pain. This will be useful information for both yourself and your therapist.

Patient _____

Therapist _____

Date _____

■ Pain   ▨ Numbness   ■ Tingling   ■ Cramp   ■ Tightness

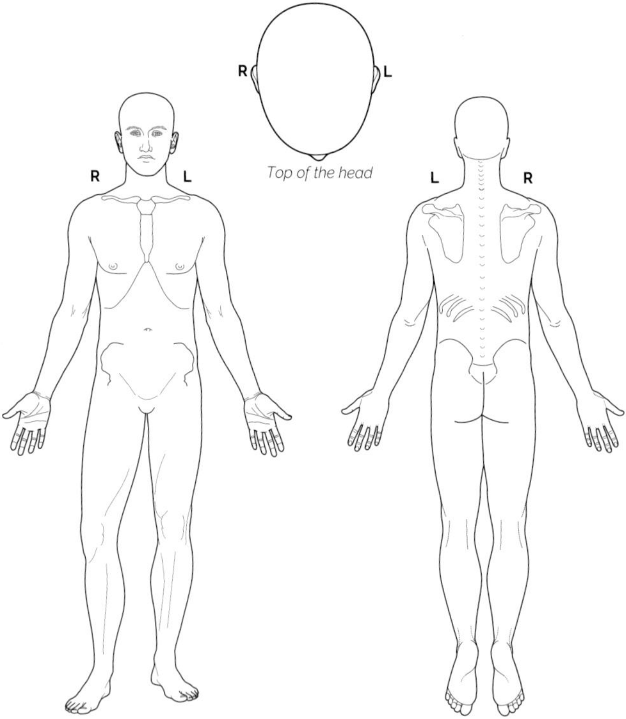

Top of the head

R   L

R   L

L   R

Patient _____

Therapist _____

Date _____

Pain   Numbness   Tingling   Cramp   Tightness

R   L

Underarm areas

Right side   *Left side*

R   L

Pubic bone

Sitting bones

Anus
Coccyx
Sacrum

Pelvic area

Schematic Interpretation of Pain Maps and Muscles Affected
(from DeLaune, V. *Pain Relief with Trigger Point Self-Help*, 2011)

Knee, Leg, Ankle, and Foot Pain

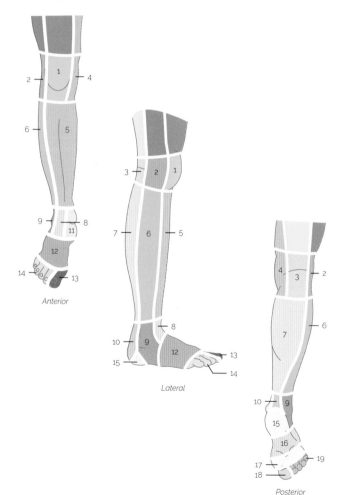

Anterior

Lateral

Posterior

1. Adductors longus & brevis

2. Vastus lateralis

3. Gastrocnemius
   Hamstring muscles
   Popliteus
   Soleus

4. Quadriceps femoris muscles
   Adductor muscles of the hip
   Sartorius

5. Tibialis anterior
   Adductors longus & brevis

6. Gastrocnemius
   Gluteus minimus
   Fibularis longus & brevis
   Vastus lateralis

7. Soleus
   Gastrocnemius
   Gluteus minimus
   Semimembranosus &
      Semitendinosus
   Flexor digitorum longus
   Tibialis posterior

8. Tibialis anterior
   Fibularis tertius
   Long extensor muscles
      of the toes

9. Fibulares

10. Soleus
    Tibialis posterior

11. Abductor hallucis
    Flexor digitorum longus

12. Extensors digitorum brevis
    and hallucis brevis
    Long extensor muscles
       of the toes
    Deep intrinsic foot muscles
    Tibialis anterior

13. Tibialis anterior
    Extensor hallucis longus
    Flexor hallucis brevis

14. Foot interossei
    Extensor digitorum longus

15. Soleus
    Quadratus plantae
    Abductor hallucis
    Tibialis posterior

16. Gastrocnemius
    Flexor digitorum longus
    Deep intrinsic foot muscles
    Soleus
    Abductor hallucis
    Tibialis posterior

17. Deep intrinsic foot muscles
    Superficial intrinsic foot
       muscles
    Long flexor muscles
       of the toes
    Tibialis posterior

18. Flexor hallucis longus
    Flexor hallucis brevis
    Tibialis posterior

19. Flexor digitorum longus
    Tibialis posterior

Lower Torso and Thigh Pain

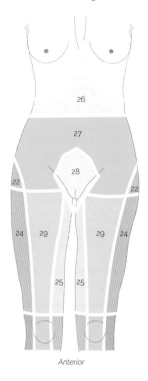

Anterior

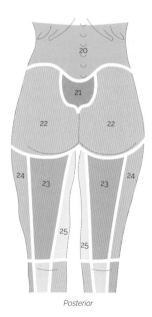

Posterior

20. Paraspinals
    Iliopsoas
    Rectus abdominis
    Gluteus medius
    Iliolumbar ligament

21. Pelvic floor
    Gluteus medius
    Quadratus lumborum
    Gluteus maximus
    Multifidi
    Rectus abdominis
    Soleus

22. Gluteus medius
    Quadratus lumborum
    Gluteus maximus
    Paraspinals
    Semitendinosus/
        Semimembranosus
    Iliolumbar ligament
    Piriformis
    Gluteus minimus
    Rectus abdominis
    Soleus
    Pelvic floor

23. Gluteus minimus
    Hamstrings
    Piriformis
    Obturator internus

24. Gluteus minimus
    Quadriceps femoris
    Piriformis
    Quadratus lumborum
    Tensor fasciae latae
    Gluteus maximus

25. Pectineus
    Vastus medialis
    Adductor muscles of the hip
    Sartorius

26. Abdominal
    Paraspinals
    Quadratus lumborum

27. Abdominal
    Paraspinals
    Quadratus lumborum

28. Pelvic floor
    Adductor magnus
    Piriformis
    Abdominal

29. Adductor muscles of the hip
    Iliopsoas
    Quadriceps femoris
    Pectineus
    Sartorius
    Quadratus lumborum
    Tensor fasciae latae

Elbow, Forearm, Wrist, and Hand Pain

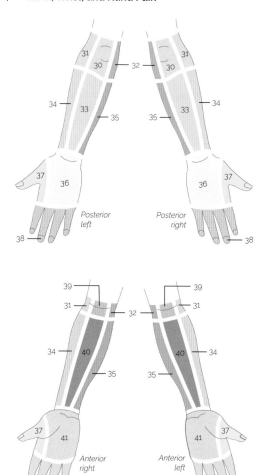

Posterior left

Posterior right

Anterior right

Anterior left

30. Triceps brachii
    Serratus posterior superior

31. Supinator
    Hand/finger extensors
    Triceps brachii/anconeus
    Supraspinatus

32. Triceps brachii
    Pectoralis major
    Pectoralis minor
    Serratus anterior
    Serratus posterior superior

33. Triceps brachii
    Teres major
    Hand/finger extensors
    Coracobrachialis
    Scalene
    Trapezius

34. Infraspinatus
    Scalene
    Brachioradialis
    Supraspinatus
    Subclavius

35. Latissimus dorsi
    Pectoralis major
    Pectoralis minor
    Serratus posterior superior

36. Hand/finger extensors
    Subscapularis
    Coracobrachialis
    Scalenes
    Latissimus dorsi
    Serratus posterior superior
    First dorsal interosseous
    Trapezius

37. Supinator
    Scalenes
    Brachialis
    Infraspinatus
    Hand/finger extensors
    Adductor/opponens pollicis
    Subclavius
    First dorsal interosseous
    Flexor pollicis longus

38. Finger extensor digitorum
    Hand interosseous
    Scalenes
    Pectoralis major
    Pectoralis minor
    Latissimus dorsi
    Subclavius

39. Brachialis
    Biceps brachii

40. Palmaris longus
    Pronator teres
    Serratus anterior
    Triceps brachii

41. Hand/finger flexors
    Opponens pollicis
    Pectoralis major
    Pectoralis minor
    Latissimus dorsi
    Palmaris longus
    Serratus anterior

42. Flexores digitorum
        superficialis and profundus
    Hand interosseous
    Latissimus dorsi
    Serratus anterior
    Subclavius

Upper Torso and Arm Pain

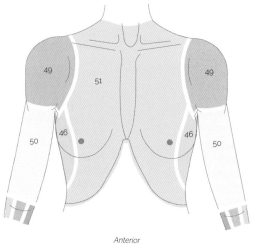

Anterior

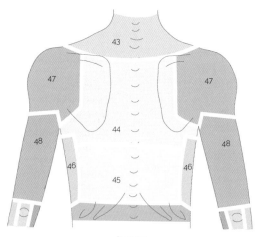

Posterior

43. Scalenes
    Levator scapulae
    Supraspinatus
    Trapezius
    Multifidi
    Rhomboids
    Splenius cervicis
    Triceps brachii
    Biceps brachii

44. Scalene
    Latissimus dorsi
    Levator scapulae
    Paraspinals
    Rhomboids
    Serratus posterior superior
    Infraspinatus
    Trapezius
    Serratus anterior
    Pectoralis major

45. Paraspinals
    Serratus posterior inferior
    Rectus abdominis
    Intercostals/diaphragm
    Latissimus dorsi
    Iliopsoas

46. Serratus anterior
    Intercostals/diaphragm
    Latissimus dorsi

47. Deltoid
    Levator scapulae
    Scalenes
    Supraspinatus
    Teres major
    Teres minor
    Subscapularis
    Serratus posterior superior
    Latissimus dorsi
    Triceps brachii
    Trapezius
    Iliocostalis thoracis

48. Scalenes
    Triceps brachii
    Deltoid
    Subscapularis
    Supraspinatus
    Teres major
    Teres minor
    Latissimus dorsi
    Serratus posterior superior
    Coracobrachialis

49. Infraspinatus
    Deltoid
    Scalenes
    Supraspinatus
    Pectoralis major/subclavius
    Pectoralis minor
    Biceps brachii
    Coracobrachialis
    Sternalis
    Latissimus dorsi

50. Scalenes
    Infraspinatus
    Biceps brachii
    Brachialis
    Triceps brachii
    Supraspinatus
    Deltoid
    Sternalis
    Subclavius

51. Pectoralis major/subclavius
    Pectoralis minor
    Scalenes
    Sternocleidomastoid
    Sternalis
    Intercostals/diaphragm
    Iliocostalis cervicis
    External oblique

Head and Neck Pain

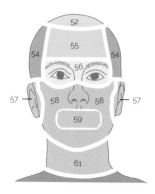 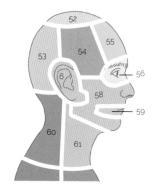

52. Sternocleidomastoid
    Splenius capitis

53. Trapezius
    Sternocleidomastoid
    Occipitalis
    Digastric
    Temporalis

54. Trapezius
    Sternocleidomastoid
    Temporalis

55. Sternocleidomastoid
    Semispinalis capitis

56. Sternocleidomastoid
    Temporalis
    Masseter
    Trapezius

57. Lateral pterygoid
    Masseter
    Sternocleidomastoid
    Medial pterygoid

58. Sternocleidomastoid
    Masseter
    Lateral pterygoid
    Trapezius
    Digastric
    Medial pterygoid

59. Temporalis
    Masseter
    Digastric

60. Trapezius
    Cervical multifidi
    Splenius cervicis
    Levator scapulae
    Infraspinatus

61. Sternocleidomastoid
    Digastric
    Medial pterygoid

CHAPTER 2

Muscles of the Face, Head, and Neck

Trigger points in the sternocleidomastoid (SCM) cause not only referred headache pain but in some cases symptoms such as dizziness (vertigo), disequilibrium, and even ringing in the ears (tinnitus). SCM trigger points can form for a variety of reasons, such as direct trauma (e.g., whiplash).

When one neck muscle develops trigger points, others can develop reflex inhibition and are forced take the strain, leading to a vicious cycle. Uneven pressure (e.g., bra straps on upper trapezius), overload from muscle contractions (e.g., neck muscles are commonly overused during abdominal exercises), and muscle imbalances in the neck, mid back, and shoulder blades (e.g., poor postural habits, such as slouched sitting or head-forward postures) are all predisposing or maintaining factors.

The relative weight of the head (10 lb/4.5 kg) changes with posture, and as we age there is a tendency toward head-forward/upper-crossed patterns, increasing the relative weight to as much as 40 lb/18 kg. Here the SCM becomes shortened and trigger points develop, which cause headaches and further limit the range of motion in rotation. The upper trapezius muscle fights against this tendency, causing trigger points to develop, which add further misery to the neck pain and headache.

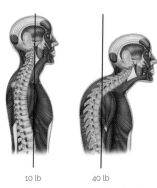

10 lb   40 lb

The relative weight of the head changes with posture.

Occipitofrontalis

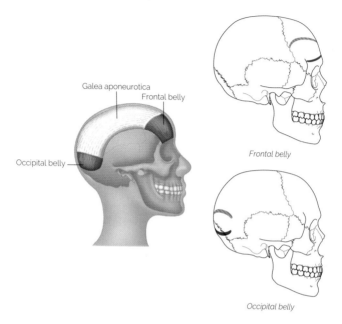

Frontal belly

Occipital belly

Latin, *frons*, forehead, front of the head; *occiput*, back of the head.

The occipitofrontalis is effectively two muscle bellies (frontal and occipital) united by an aponeurosis called the *galea aponeurotica*, so named because it forms what resembles a helmet (Latin *galea*).

Origin
Frontal belly: skin of eyebrows.
Occipital belly: lateral two-thirds of superior nuchal line of occipital bone. Mastoid process of temporal bone.

Insertion
Galea aponeurotica.

Nerve
Facial nerve (VII) (posterior auricular and temporal branches).

Action
Frontal belly: raises eyebrows and wrinkles skin of forehead horizontally.
Occipital belly: pulls scalp backward.

Basic Functional Movement
Facilitates facial expressions, e.g., looking surprised/frowning.

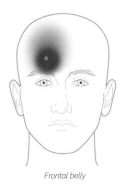

Frontal belly

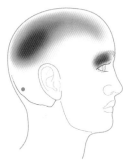

Occipital belly

Referred Pain Patterns

Frontal belly: localized pain with some referral upward and over forehead on same side.
Occipital belly: pain in lateral and anterior scalp; diffuse into back of head and into orbit.

Indications

Headache, pain (back of head), cannot sleep on back/pillow, earache, pain behind eye/eyebrow/eyelid, visual activity, "jumping text" on reading black and white print, squinting, wrinkly forehead, tension headache, pain above eye.

Causes

Anxiety, overwork, lifestyle, computer use, wrong glasses, frowning.

Differential Diagnosis

Scalp tingling. Greater occipital nerve entrapment.

Connections

Suboccipital muscles, clavicular division of SCM, semispinalis capitis, zygomaticus major, platysma, scalenes, posterior neck muscles, eye muscles.

Orbicularis Oculi

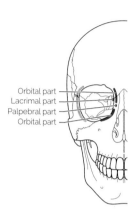

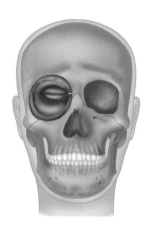

Orbital part
Lacrimal part
Palpebral part
Orbital part

Latin, *orbiculus*, small circular disc; *oculus*, eye.

This complex and extremely important muscle consists of three parts—orbital (circling the eye), palpebral (in eyelids, **Latin**, *palpebra*, eyelid), and lacrimal (behind medial palpebral ligament and lacrimal sac, **Latin**, *lacrima*, tear); together they form an important protective mechanism surrounding the eye.

Origin
Orbital part: frontal bone. Frontal process of maxilla. Medial palpebral ligament.
Palpebral part: medial palpebral ligament.
Lacrimal part: lacrimal bone.

Insertion
Orbital part: circular path around orbit, returning to origin.
Palpebral part: lateral palpebral raphe.
Lacrimal part: lateral palpebral raphe.

Nerve
Facial nerve (VII) (temporal and zygomatic branches).

Action
Orbital part: strongly closes eyelids (firmly "screws up" eye).
Palpebral part: gently closes eyelids (and comes into action involuntarily, as in blinking).
Lacrimal part: dilates lacrimal sac and brings lacrimal canals onto surface of eye.

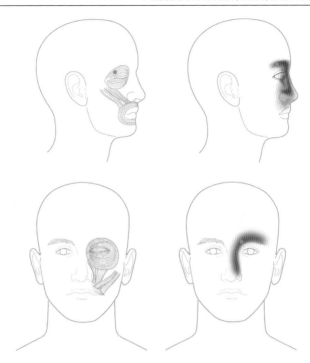

Referred Pain Patterns

Palpebral: localized "searing" pain above eye and up to ipsilateral nostril.

Lacrimal: into eye, sinus pain, bridge of nose pain. Ice cream often reproduces eye pain/headache.

Indications

Headache, migraine, trigeminal neuralgia, eyestrain, "twitching" eyes, poor eyesight, drooping eyelid, sinus pain, eyebrow pain, dry eyes.

Causes

Eyesight problems, anxiety, frowning, tension, computer screen overuse.

Differential Diagnosis

Ptosis—Horner's syndrome.

Connections

Digastric, temporalis, trapezius, spleneii, posterior cervical muscles. Often associated with SCM.

Corrugator Supercilii

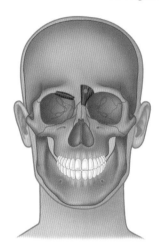

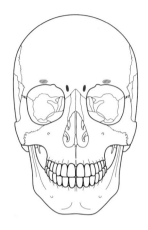

Latin, *corrugare*, to wrinkle up; *supercilii*, of the eyebrow.

Origin
Medial end of superciliary arch of frontal bone.

Insertion
Deep surface of skin under medial half of eyebrows.

Nerve
Facial nerve (VII) (temporal branch).

Action
Draws eyebrows medially and downward, thus producing vertical wrinkles.

Basic Functional Movement
Frowning.

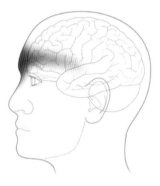

Referred Pain Patterns
Medial eyebrow zone.

Indications
Headache, eyebrow pain.

Causes
The corrugator and frontalis muscles are often

activated together by people who constantly frown. Psychological stress. The corrugator particularly may entrap the supraorbital nerve.

Differential Diagnosis
Supraorbital nerve entrapment.

Connections
Frontalis muscle, procerus. Local facial muscles.

Procerus

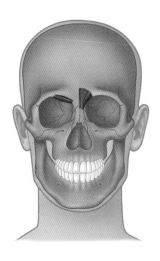
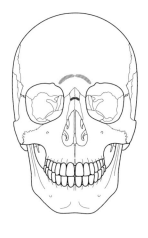

Latin, *procerus*, long.

Origin
Fascia over nasal bone. Upper part of lateral nasal cartilage.

Insertion
Skin between eyebrows.

Nerve
Facial nerve (VII) (temporal branch).

Action
Produces transverse wrinkles over bridge of nose. Pulls medial portion of eyebrows downward.

Basic Functional Movement
Enables strong "sniffing" and sneezing.

Referred Pain Patterns
Small patch locally at the medial edge of the brow.

Indications
Eye strain, frowning pain, localized headache on frowning, migraine.

Causes
Psychological stress, eye strain, computer and phone screen overuse, frowning, squinting.

Differential Diagnosis
Supraorbital nerve entrapment, frontalis headache.

Connections
The procerus and corrugator muscles are implicated in migraine headache. Local facial muscles.

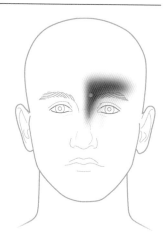

Buccinator

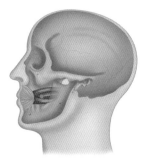

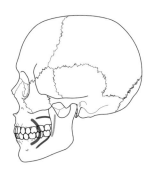

Latin, *bucca*, cheek.

Forms the substance of the cheek.

Origin
Posterior parts of maxilla and mandible; pterygomandibular raphe.

Insertion
Blends with orbicularis oris and into lips.

Nerve
Facial nerve (VII) (buccal branch).

Action
Presses cheek against teeth.
Compresses distended cheeks.

Referred Pain Patterns
Local dental and upper gum
pain.

Indications
Main muscle of the cheek, TPs
mostly mid-cheek, between angle
of mouth and ramus of mandible.

Causes
Chewing, frowning, habitual
facial expressions, tics, dental
work, dental appliances.
Hyperventilation syndrome.

Differential Diagnosis
Blepherospasm. The parotid
duct pierces the buccinator in the
region of the third molar.

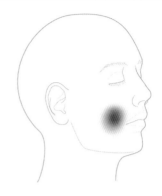

Connections
Orbicularis oris, larger local
muscle trigger points in neck and
shoulder muscles. Local facial
muscles.

Zygomaticus Major

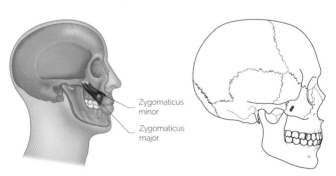

Zygomaticus
minor

Zygomaticus
major

Greek, *zygoma*, bar, bolt.
Latin, *major*, larger.

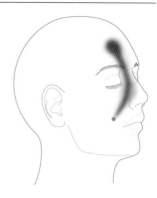

Origin
Posterior part of lateral surface of zygomatic bone.

Insertion
Skin at corner of mouth.

Nerve
Facial nerve (VII) (zygomatic and buccal branches).

Action
Pulls corner of mouth upward and laterally, as in smiling.

Basic Functional Movement
Smiling.

Referred Pain Patterns
2 cm patch on forehead, streaking laterally to the nose and into the cheek.

Indications
Cheek pain, headache, TMJ, hemifacial pain, can become intractable.

Causes
Prolonged dental work, post-tic douloureux, smiling too much!

Differential Diagnosis
Dental issues. Myalgia. Neuromuscular diseases. Lacerations. Contusions. Bell's palsy. Infectious myositis and myopathy. Trigeminal neuralgia—tic douloureux.

Connections
Lateral pterygoid, orbicularis oculi, masseter.

Masseter

Greek, *maseter*, chewer.

The masseter is the most superficial muscle of mastication, easily felt when the jaw is clenched.

Origin
Zygomatic arch and maxillary process of zygomatic bone.

Insertion
Lateral surface of ramus of mandible.

Nerve
Trigeminal nerve (V) (mandibular division).

Action
Elevation of mandible.

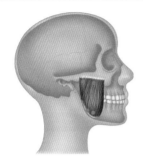
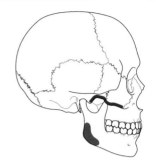

Basic Functional Movement
Chewing food.

Referred Pain Patterns
Superficial: eyebrow, maxilla, and mandible (anterior). Upper and lower molar teeth.
Deep: ear and TMJ.

Indications
Trismus (severely restricted jaw), TMJ pain, tension/stress headache, ear pain, ipsilateral tinnitus, dental pain, bruxism, sinusitis pain, puffiness under

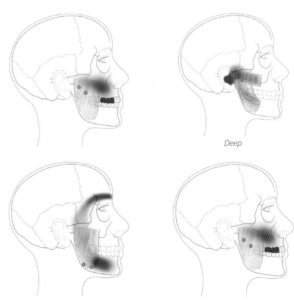

Deep

Superficial

the eyes (often present in singers).

Causes
Chewing gum, tooth grinding/ bruxism, prolonged dental work, stress, emotional tension, head-forward postures, occupation.

Differential Diagnosis
TMJ pain/syndrome. Tinnitus. Trismus.

Connections
Ipsilateral temporalis, medial pterygoid, contralateral masseter, SCM.

Temporalis

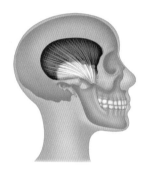
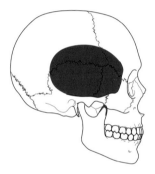

Latin, *temporalis*, of time.

Temporalis is a broad fan-shaped muscle and covers much of the temporal bone.

Origin
Bone of temporal fossa. Temporal fascia.

Insertion
Coronoid process of mandible. Anterior margin of ramus of mandible.

Nerve
Anterior and posterior deep temporal nerves from the trigeminal nerve (V) (mandibular division).

Action
Elevation and retraction of mandible.

Basic Functional Movement
Chewing food.

Referred Pain Patterns

Upper incisors and supraorbital ridge. Maxillary teeth and mid-temple pain. TMJ and mid-temple pain. Localized (backward and upward).

Indications

Headache, toothache, TMJ syndrome, hypersensitivity of teeth, prolonged dental work, eyebrow pain, headaches, bruxism, sinusitis pain, trismus (lockjaw), tingling in cheek area.

Causes

Chewing gum, tooth grinding/ bruxism, prolonged dental work, stress, emotional tension, jaw/ bite alignment, nail biting, thumb sucking.

Differential Diagnosis

Temporalis tendinitis. Polymyalgia rheumatica. Temporal arteritis, or giant cell arteritis (GCA).

Connections

Upper trapezius, SCM, masseter.

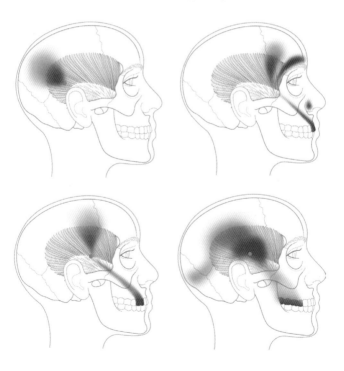

Lateral Pterygoid

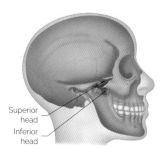

Superior head
Inferior head

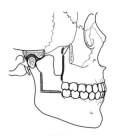

Greek, *pterygoeides*, wing-like. **Latin**, *lateralis*, relating to the side.

The superior head of this muscle is sometimes called *sphenomeniscus*, because it inserts into the disc of the temporomandibular joint.

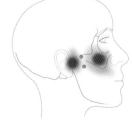

Origin
Superior head: roof of infratemporal fossa.
Inferior head: lateral surface of lateral plate of pterygoid process.

Insertion
Superior head: capsule and articular disc of temporomandibular joint.
Inferior head: neck of mandible.

Nerve
Trigeminal nerve (V) (mandibular division).

Action
Protrusion and side-to-side movements of mandible, as in chewing.

Basic Functional Movement
Chewing food.

Referred Pain Patterns
Two zones of pain:
(1) TMJ in a 1 cm localized zone;
(2) zygomatic arch in a 3–4 cm zone.

Indications
TMJ syndrome, cranio-mandibular pain, problems chewing/masticating, tinnitus, sinusitis, decreased jaw opening, headaches, bruxism, sinusitis pain, trismus (lockjaw), tingling in cheek area.

Causes
Chewing gum, tooth grinding/
bruxism, prolonged dental work,
stress, emotional tension, jaw/
bite alignment, nail biting, thumb
sucking.

Connections
TMJ, atlanto-occipital joint facets,
neck muscles, masseter, medial
pterygoid, temporalis (anterior),
zygomaticus, buccinator,
orbicularis oculi, SCM.

Differential Diagnosis
Arthritic TMJ. Anatomical
variations of TMJ. Tic douloureux
(trigeminal neuralgia). Shingles.

Medial Pterygoid

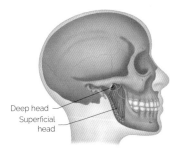
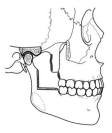

Deep head
Superficial
head

Greek, *pterygoeides*, wing-like.
Latin, *medialis*, relating to the
middle.

This muscle mirrors the masseter
muscle in both its position and
action, with the ramus of the
mandible positioned between the
two muscles.

Origin
Deep head: medial surface
of lateral pterygoid plate of
pterygoid process. Pyramidal
process of palatine bone.

Superficial head: tuberosity of
maxilla and pyramidal process of
palatine bone.

Insertion
Medial surface of ramus and
angle of mandible.

Nerve
Trigeminal nerve (V)
(mandibular division).

Action
Elevation and side-to-side
movement of mandible, as in
chewing.

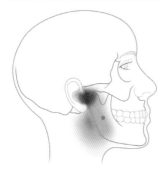

Deep head

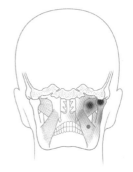

Superficial head

Basic Functional Movement
Chewing food.

Referred Pain Patterns
Localized zone about TMJ radiating broadly down ramus of jaw toward the clavicle.

Indications
Pain in throat, mouth, and pharynx, odynophagia, TMJ syndrome, lockjaw, inability to fully open jaw, ENT pain, excessive dental treatment, TMJ pain on biting, bruxism, blocked ears.

Causes
Chewing gum, tooth grinding/ bruxism, prolonged dental work, stress, emotional tension, jaw/ bite alignment, nail biting, thumb sucking, incorrect pillows.

Differential Diagnosis
TMJ syndrome. ENT pathologies. GI referral, e.g., Barrett's syndrome (esophagus). Bruxism.

Connections
Masseter, temporalis, lateral pterygoid, tongue, SCM, digastric, longus capitis/ colli, platysma, clavipectoral fascia, zygomaticus, buccinator, tensor vali palentini, salpingopharyngeus, SCM.

Platysma

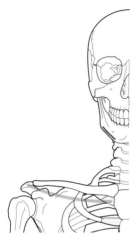 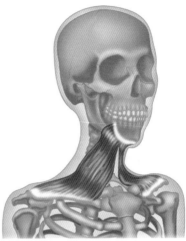

Greek, *platys*, broad, flat.

This muscle may be seen to stand out in a runner finishing a hard race.

Origin
Subcutaneous fascia of upper quarter of chest (i.e., fascia overlying pectoralis major and deltoid muscles).

Insertion
Subcutaneous fascia and muscles of chin and jaw. Inferior border of mandible.

Nerve
Facial nerve (VII) (cervical branch).

Action
Pulls lower lip from corner of mouth downward and laterally. Draws skin of chest upward.

Basic Functional Movement
Produces expression of being startled or of sudden fright.

Referred Pain Patterns
Cheek, chin, mandible. Directly on or above clavicle.

Indications
Pricking sensation or hemifacial pain on lateral face and ipsilateral inferior ramus mandible. TPs usually found over SCM, clavicular TPs may refer hot prickling across front of chest.

Causes
Postural, facial pain during expression (horror and surprise), tics, gurning, age, genetics.

Differential Diagnosis
Look into postural maladaptations, facial nerve (VII) injury.

Connections
SCM and scalene muscles.

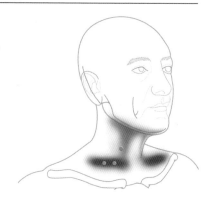

Digastric

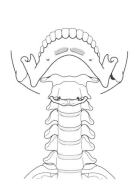

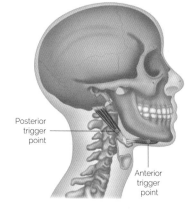

Posterior trigger point

Anterior trigger point

Latin, *digastricus*, having two (muscle) bellies.

Origin
Anterior belly: digastric fossa on inner side of lower border of mandible.

Posterior belly: mastoid notch on medial side of mastoid process of temporal bone.

Insertion
Body of hyoid bone via a fascial sling over an intermediate tendon.

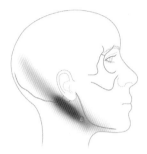

Posterior trigger point

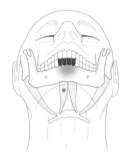

Anterior trigger point

Nerve
Anterior belly: mylohyoid nerve, from trigeminal V nerve (mandibular division).
Posterior belly: facial nerve (VII) (digastric branch).

Action
Anterior belly: raises hyoid bone. Opens mouth by lowering mandible.
Posterior belly: pulls hyoid upward and back.

Referred Pain Patterns
Anterior: lower four incisor teeth, tongue, and lip, occasionally to chin.
Posterior: strong 2 cm zone around mastoid and vaguely the zone to chin and throat, occasionally to scalp.

Indications
Throat pain, dental pain (four lower incisors), headache, jaw pain, renal tubular acidosis, prolonged/extensive dental work (blurred vision and dizziness), lower mouth opening, difficulty swallowing, vocal/singing problems.

Causes
Head-forward/upper crossed pattern, poor bite mechanics and/or clenching/grinding of teeth (bruxism), whiplash, telephone to chin, musical instruments (e.g., violin or wind instruments).

Differential Diagnosis
Dental problems—malocclusion. Hyoid bone. Thyroid problems. Thymus gland. Sinusitis. Carotid artery.

Connections
SCM, sternothyroid, mylohyoid, stylohyoid, longus colli/capitis, geniohyoid, cervical vertebrae, temporalis, masseter.

Omohyoid

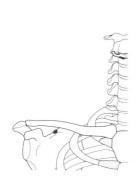

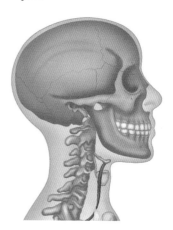

Greek, *omos*, shoulder; *hyoeides*, shaped like the Greek letter upsilon (υ).

Origin
Inferior belly: upper border of scapula medial to the scapular notch.
Superior belly: intermediate tendon.

Insertion
Inferior belly: intermediate tendon.
Superior belly: lower border of hyoid bone, lateral to insertion of sternohyoid.

Note: The intermediate tendon is tied down to the clavicle and first rib by a sling of the cervical fascia.

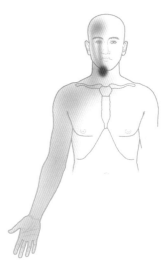

Nerve
Ventral rami of C1 to C3 through ansa cervicalis.

Action
Depresses and fixes hyoid bone.

Referred Pain Patterns
Small patch around muscle, and radiating into lateral mandible, forehead, shoulder, arm, and into hand.

Indications
Function in pairs, tongue-related pain, moving tip of tongue around mouth and sticking tongue out. Pressure on brachial plexus.

Causes
Tongue-tie, hyperventilation, smoking, dysphagia, first rib syndromes.

Differential Diagnosis
Hemifacial paralysis, stroke, burning tongue.

Connections
One of the infrahyoid group (all attached proximally to the hyoid bone).

Longus Colli

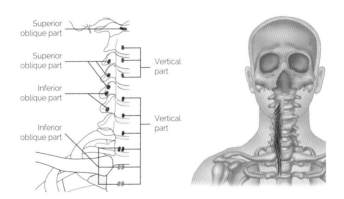

Superior oblique part
Superior oblique part
Inferior oblique part
Inferior oblique part
Vertical part
Vertical part

Latin, *longus*, long; *colli*, of the neck.

Longus colli can be divided into three parts—superior oblique, inferior oblique, and vertical—and is the largest member of the prevertebral muscles.

Origin
Superior oblique: transverse processes of C3–5.
Inferior oblique: anterior surface of bodies of T1, 2, maybe T3.
Vertical: anterior surface of bodies of T1–3 and C5–7.

57

Insertion

Superior oblique: anterior arch of atlas.
Inferior oblique: transverse processes of C5–6.
Vertical: transverse processes of C2–4.

Nerve

Ventral rami of cervical nerves C2–6.

Action

Flexes neck anteriorly and laterally and slight rotation to opposite side.

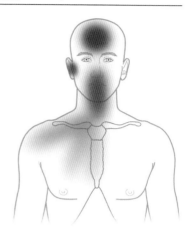

Basic Functional Movement

Gives control and quality of movement to neck flexion.

Referred Pain Patterns

Pain map is large involving face, throat and upper chest. Often vague or nonspecific.

Indications

Anterior cervicalgia, facial pain. Pain across the upper chest on the affected side to the ipsilateral deltoid, a feeling of tightness across the chest, local pain is reported as a deep, thin, and acute sensation at the vertebral level, rising up to the eye on the ipsilateral side.

Causes

Whiplash associated disorder (WAD); longus colli bilaterally decelerates extension of the neck, and unilaterally decelerates ipsilateral rotation and lateral neck extension. Occupational- and sports-related (inappropriate) neck movements. Cervical disc disease with loss of cervical lordosis.

Differential Diagnosis

Cervical disc disease. Whiplash associated disorder (WAD), thyroid pathology, parathyroid pathology, facet disease.

Connections

Longus colli and associated anterior muscles of the neck. Sternocleidomastoid pain issues.

Longus Capitis

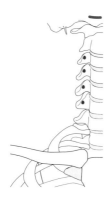

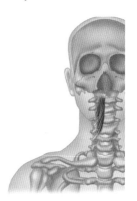

Latin, *longus*, long; *capitis*, of the head.

Longus capitis lies anterior to the superior oblique fibers of longus colli.

Origin
Transverse processes of third to sixth cervical vertebrae (C3–6).

Insertion
Inferior surface of basilar part of occipital bone.

Nerve
Ventral rami of cervical nerves C1–3, (C4).

Action
Flexes head.

Basic Functional Movement
Gives control and quality of movement to neck flexion.

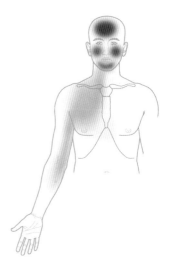

Referred Pain Patterns
Specific pain patterns are not reported in the literature but believed to cause pain to the laryngeal region, anterior neck and sometimes into the mouth.

Indications
Anterior neck pain.

Causes
Postural, whiplash associated disorder (WAD), ill-fitting glasses, neck brace, upper crossed posture, age related cervical disorders. Loss of cervical lordosis.

Differential Diagnosis
Cervical disc disease, thyroid pathology, parathyroid pathology, facet disease.

Connections
Longus colli and anterior vertebral muscles. SCM pain issues.

Scalenes

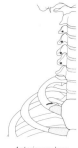

Anterior scalene

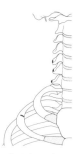

Posterior scalene

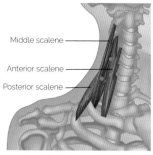

Middle scalene ——————
Anterior scalene ——————
Posterior scalene ——————

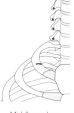

Middle scalene

Greek, *skalenos*, uneven.
Latin, *anterior*, at the front; *medius*, middle; *posterior*, at the back.

Origin
Anterior: anterior tubercles of transverse processes of third to sixth cervical vertebrae (C3–6).

Middle: transverse processes of C2–7.
Posterior: posterior tubercles of transverse processes of C4–6.

Insertion
Anterior: scalene tubercle and upper surface of first rib.
Middle: upper surface of first rib, behind groove for subclavian artery.
Posterior: upper surface of second rib.

Nerve
Anterior: ventral rami of cervical nerves C4–7.
Middle: ventral rami of cervical nerves C3–7.
Posterior: ventral rami of lower cervical nerves C5–7.

Action
Acting on both sides: flex neck; raise first or second rib during active respiratory inhalation.
Acting on one side: side flexes and rotates head.

Basic Functional Movement
Primarily a muscle of inspiration.

Referred Pain Patterns
Anterior: persistent aching, pectoralis region to the nipple.
Middle: front and back of the arm to the thumb and index finger.
Posterior: upper medial border of scapula.

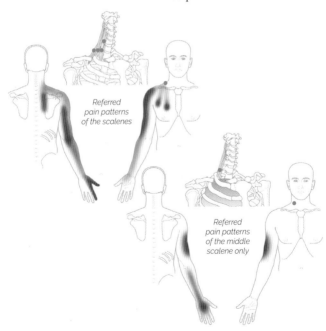

Referred pain patterns of the scalenes

Referred pain patterns of the middle scalene only

Indications
Back/shoulder/arm pain,
thoracic outlet syndrome, scalene
syndrome, edema in the hand,
phantom limb pain, asthma,
chronic lung disease, whiplash,
"restless neck," irritability,
hyperventilation syndrome,
panic attacks.

Causes
Anxiety, stress, pillow height,
chronic lung problems, smoking,
heavy lifting/bracing, allergies,
wind instruments, RTA.

Differential Diagnosis
Brachial plexus. Subclavian
vessels. Cervical discs (C5–6).
Thoracic outlet syndrome.
Angina. Carpal tunnel syndrome.
Upper trapezius. SCM. Splenius
capitis.

Connections
SCM, levator scapulae, platysma.

Sternocleidomastoid

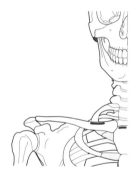 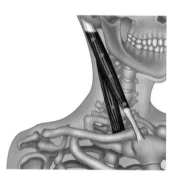

Greek, *sternon*, chest; *kleis*, key;
mastoeides, breast shaped.

This muscle is a long strap
muscle with two heads. It is
sometimes injured at birth, and
may be partly replaced by fibrous
tissue that contracts to produce a
torticollis (wry neck).

Origin
Sternal head: upper part of
anterior surface of manubrium
of sternum.
Clavicular head: upper surface
of medial third of clavicle.

Insertion
Sternal head: lateral one-half of
superior nuchal line of occipital
bone.
Clavicular head: outer surface of
mastoid process of temporal bone.

Nerve
Accessory nerve (XI) and
branches from ventral rami of
cervical nerves C2, 3 (C4).

Action

Bilateral contraction: draws head forward (protracts); raises sternum, and consequently ribs, during deep inhalation.
Unilateral contraction: flexes head to same side; rotates head to opposite side.

Basic Functional Movement

Examples: turning the head to look over the shoulder, raising the head from a pillow.

Referred Pain Patterns

Sternal head: pain in occiput, radiating anteriorly to eyebrow, cheek, and throat (eye and sinus).
Clavicular head: frontal headache, earache, mastoid pain (dizziness and spatial awareness).

Indications

Tension headache, whiplash, stiff neck, atypical facial neuralgia, hangover headache, postural dizziness, altered SNS symptoms to half of face, lowered spatial awareness, ptosis. Associated with (existing) persistent dry, tickling cough, sinusitis and chronic sore throats, increased eye tearing and reddening, popping sounds in the ear (one sided), balance problems, and veering to one side when driving.

Causes

Anxiety, stress, pillow height, allergies, weight lifting, RTA, car sickness, trauma, incorrect swimming styles, tight shirt collars, work posture and ergonomics.

Differential Diagnosis

Trigeminal neuralgia. Facial neuralgia. Vestibulocochlear problems. Lymphadenopathy. Levator scapulae. Upper trapezius. Splenius capitis.

Connections

Trapezius, masseter, platysma, scalenes, levator scapulae, sternalis, temporalis, pectoralis major.

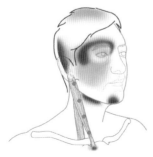

Sternal head

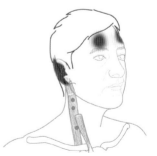

Clavicular head

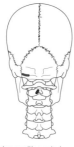

Rectus capitis posterior major

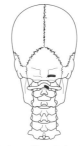

Rectus capitis posterior minor

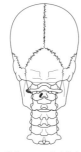

Obliquus capitis inferior

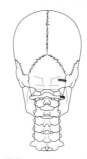

Obliquus capitis superior

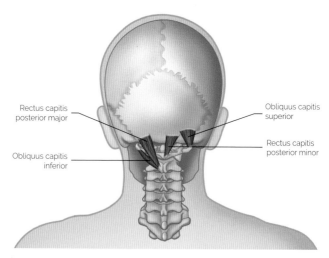

Rectus capitis
posterior major

Obliquus capitis superior

Rectus capitis
posterior minor

Obliquus capitis
inferior

Suboccipital Group

The suboccipital group of muscles lies deep in the neck, anterior to semispinalis capitis, longissimus capitis, and splenius capitis. The muscle group encloses a triangular space known as the **suboccipital triangle**.

Rectus Capitis Posterior Major

Latin, *rectus*, straight; *capitis*, of the head; *posterior*, at the back; *major*, larger.

Origin
Spinous process of axis.

Insertion
Lateral portion of occipital bone below inferior nuchal line.

Nerve
Suboccipital nerve (dorsal ramus of first cervical nerve C1).

Action
Extends head. Rotates head to same side.

Basic Functional Movement
Helps control the act of looking upward and over the shoulder.

Rectus Capitis Posterior Minor

Latin, *rectus*, straight; *capitis*, of the head; *posterior*, at the back; *minor*, smaller.

Origin
Posterior tubercle of atlas.

Insertion
Medial portion of occipital bone below inferior nuchal line.

Nerve
Suboccipital nerve (dorsal ramus of first cervical nerve C1).

Action
Extends head.

Basic Functional Movement
Helps control the act of looking upward.

Obliquus Capitis Inferior

Latin, *obliquus*, diagonal, slanted; *capitis*, of the head; *inferior*, lower.

Origin
Spinous process of axis.

Insertion
Transverse process of atlas.

Nerve
Suboccipital nerve (dorsal ramus of first cervical nerve C1).

Action
Rotates atlas upon axis, thereby rotating head to same side.

Basic Functional Movement
Gives stability to the head when it is turned.

Obliquus Capitis Superior

Latin, *obliquus*, diagonal, slanted; *capitis*, of the head; *superior*, upper.

Origin
Transverse process of atlas.

Insertion
Occipital bone between superior and inferior nuchal lines.

Nerve
Suboccipital nerve (dorsal ramus of first cervical nerve C1).

Action
Extends head and flexes to the same side.

Basic Functional Movement
Helps control the act of looking upward.

Referred Pain Patterns
Deep local pain in suboccipital region, radiating caudally and ventrally. Retrobulbar neuritis pain.

Indications
Pain shooting from the back of the head into the eye, temple headache (particularly migraine), greater occipital neuralgia (GON).

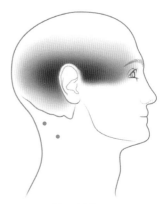

Suboccipital group

Causes
Occupational ergonomics, ill-fitting glasses, eye strain, overuse of computer and cell-phone screens, sleeping position, scoliosis, whiplash-associated disorder (WAD).

Differential Diagnosis
Retrobulbar neuritis. Migraine. GON. Cervicogenic headache. Splenius cervicis. Occipitofrontalis. Upper trapezius.

Connections
Suboccipital muscles, splenius cervicis, longissimus capitis.

Trigger Points and Headaches

Headaches can be roughly divided into three categories: Tension type headache (TTH), cervicogenic headache (referred pain from the neck, CGH), and migraines.

Here are some key muscles to consider:

TTH: Trapezius, SCM, temporalis, masseter, and occipitofrontalis.

CGH: Splenius capitis and cervicis, suboccipitals, and longus colli.

TMJ: Temporalis, masseter, lateral pterygoid.

The presence of trigger points in neck and shoulder muscles may be a part of the triggering and/or maintaining mechanisms via the

nociceptive drive to the dorsal horn. It is worth noting that the caudate nucleus of the trigeminal nerve (thought to be connected to migraines) often extends to C5 in the neck.

TMJ: Pain at the temples/in front of the ears.

Sinusitis: Pain behind the brow bone and/or cheekbones.

Cluster: Pain in and around one eye.

Tension: Pain is like a band squeezing the head.

Migraine: Pain (one sided), nausea, and visual changes.

Cervicogenic: Pain at the top and/or back of the head.

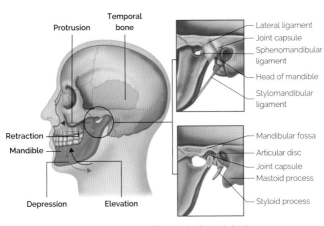

The temporomandibular joint (lateral view).

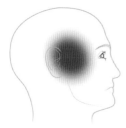

Temporomandibular joint (TMJ)
Pain at the temples, in front of the ears

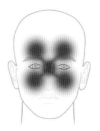

Sinusitis
Pain behind the brow bone and/or cheekbones

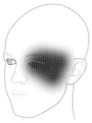

Cluster
Pain in and around one eye

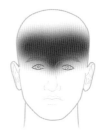

Tension
Pain like a band squeezing the head

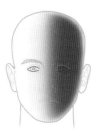

Migraine
Pain (one sided), nausea and visual changes

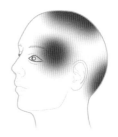

Cervicogenic (referred from the neck)
Pain at the top and/or back of the head

CHAPTER 3

Muscles of the Trunk and Spine

As with the neck, lifestyle factors often predispose to or maintain trigger points in the spine and trunk. These factors include a poor posture held for too long (e.g., sleeping postures, see page 22; occupational postures, such as sitting with the head rotated to one side or incorrect ergonomics—e.g., using a computer screen at the wrong angle or with copy to the side, see page 23), and mental and emotional stress.

Trigger points rarely occur in isolation, and there is often a push-pull relationship between agonists, antagonists, and fixators. A common site of trigger points in the spine is the trapezius. Due to its shape and position, it often has to withstand pressure from a weight (e.g., a shoulder bag) and is susceptible to whiplash. Also consider the rhomboids and pectoralis major.

Trigger points in the erector spinae can elicit pain over the whole back, with pain emanating into the lumbo-pelvic, chest, and abdominal regions.

Low back pain is considered one of the most common pain disorders. Acute low back pain responds well to trigger point therapy, but chronic pain is more problematic, with up to twelve muscle groups involved. However, four muscles that are implicated in nearly all cases of low back pain are quadratus lumborum, gluteus medius, iliopsoas, and rectus abdominis.

Erector Spinae (Sacrospinalis)

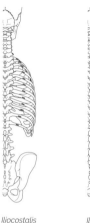

Iliocostalis thoracis

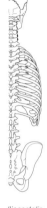

Iliocostalis cervicis

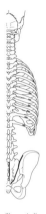

Iliocostalis lumborum

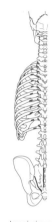

Longissimus thoracis

Latin, *erector*, one who builds, *spinae*, of the spine.

Three sets of muscles organized in parallel columns. From lateral to medial, they are: iliocostalis, longissimus, and spinalis.

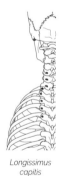

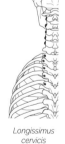

Longissimus capitis

Longissimus cervicis

Origin
Slips of muscle arising from the sacrum. Iliac crest. Spinous and transverse processes of vertebrae. Ribs.

Insertion
Ribs. Transverse and spinous processes of vertebrae. Occipital bone.

Nerve
Dorsal rami of cervical, thoracic, and lumbar spinal nerves.

Action
Extends and laterally flexes vertebral column (i.e., bending backward and sideways). Helps maintain correct curvature of spine in the erect and sitting positions. Steadies the vertebral column on the pelvis during walking.

Basic Functional Movement

Keeps back straight (with correct curvatures), therefore maintains posture.

Referred Pain Patterns

Thoracic spine—iliocostalis: medially toward the spine, and anteriorly toward the abdomen.
Lumbar spine—iliocostalis: mid buttock.
Thoracic spine—iliocostalis: buttock and sacroiliac area. Spinalis displays the same referred pain patterns as multifidus.

Indications

Low back pain (esp. after lifting), reduced ROM in the spine, low back pain, low grade back ache worsening toward the end of the day.

Causes

Poor posture, playing musical instruments, lying on front with head propped up, poor glasses, upper crossed pattern, kyphosis, scoliosis, wear and tear, cold drafts/air conditioning, vertebral alignment issues, certain sports (e.g., archery), tight shirt/tie, depression.

Differential Diagnosis

Angina. Visceral pain. Radiculopathy. Ligamentous, discogenic, sacroiliac. Piriformis. Pathological: aortic aneurysm. Visceral pathology. Space-occupying lesion. Pelvic inflammatory disease.

Connections

Pectoralis major.

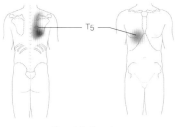

Iliocostalis thoracis

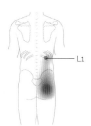

Iliocostalis lumborum

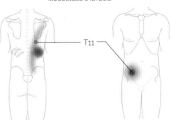

Iliocostalis thoracis

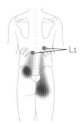

Longissimus thoracis

Posterior Cervical Muscles

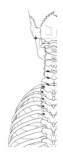
Longissimus capitis

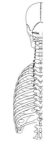
Semispinalis capitis

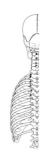
Semispinalis cervicis

Latin, *longissimus*, longest; *capitis*, of the head; *semispinalis*, half spinal; *cervicis*, of the neck.

Origin
Longissimus capitis: transverse processes of T1–5. Articular processes of C5–7.
Semispinalis cervicis: transverse processes of T1–6.
Semispinalis capitis: transverse processes of C4–T7.

Insertion
Longissimus capitis: posterior part of mastoid process of temporal bone.
Semispinalis cervicis: spinous processes of C2–5.
Semispinalis capitis: between superior and inferior nuchal lines of occipital bone.

Nerve
Longissimus capitis: dorsal rami of middle and lower cervical nerves.
Semispinalis cervicis: dorsal rami of thoracic and cervical nerves.
Semispinalis capitis: dorsal rami of cervical nerves.

Action
Longissimus capitis: extends and rotates head. Helps maintain correct curvature of thoracic and cervica spine in the erect and sitting positions.
Semispinalis cervicis: extends thoracic and cervical parts of vertebral column. Assists rotation of thoracic and cervical vertebrae.
Semispinalis capitis: most powerful extensor of the head. Assists in rotation of head.

Basic Functional Movement
Longissimus capitis: keeps upper back straight (with correct curvatures).
Semispinalis cervicis and capitis.
Examples: looking up; turning head to look behind.

Referred Pain Patterns
Several areas along the fibers, all radiating superiorly into head and skull and toward frontal region.

Indications
Headache, neck pain and stiffness, decreased cervical flexion, suboccipital pain, restricted neck rotation (often related to prolonged occupational positions), whiplash, pain using certain pillows, "burning" in scalp.

Causes
Poor posture, playing musical instruments, lying on front with head propped up, poor glasses, upper crossed pattern, kyphosis, scoliosis, wear and tear, cold drafts/air conditioning, vertebral alignment issues, certain sports (e.g., archery), tight shirt/tie, depression.

Differential Diagnosis
Cervical mechanical dysfunction. Spondyloarthropathy of facets. Vertebral artery syndrome. Discopathy (cervical) first rib dysfunction. Polymyalgia rheumatica. Rheumatoid arthritis. Osteoarthritis. Ankylosing spondylitis. Paget's disease. Psoriatic arthropathy.

Connections
Trapezius, erector spinae, temporalis, digastric, infraspinatus, levator scapulae, SCM, splenius capitis/cervicis, suboccipital muscles, occipitalis, pectoralis major.

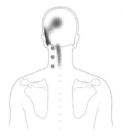

Longissimus capitis

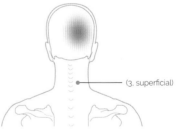

Semispinalis capitis (middle) and cervicis (3, superficial)

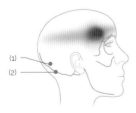

Semispinalis capitis (upper) (1) (2)

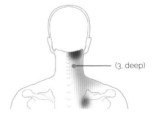

Multifidi (mid cervical) (3, deep)

Multifidus and Rotatores

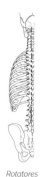

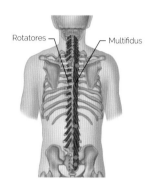

Rotatores — — Multifidus

Rotatores

Multifidus

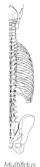

Multifidus

Latin, *multi*, many; *findere*, to split.

Part of the transversospinales group that lies in the furrow between the spines of the vertebrae and their transverse processes. Multifidus lies deep to semispinalis and erector spinae.

Origin
Sacrum, origin of erector spinae, posterior superior iliac spine, mammillary processes (posterior borders of superior articular processes) of L1–5. Transverse processes of T1–12. Articular processes of L4–7.

Insertion
Base of spinous processes of L5–C2.

Nerve
Dorsal rami of spinal nerves.

Action
Gives individual vertebral joints control during movement by the more powerful superficial prime movers. Extension, side flexion, and rotation of vertebral column.

Rotatores

Latin, *rota*, wheel.

Deepest layer of the transversospinales group.

Origin
Transverse process of each vertebra.

Insertion
Base of spinous process of adjoining vertebra above.

Nerve
Dorsal rami of spinal nerves.

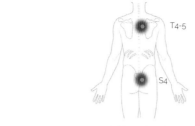

Multifidus and rotatores

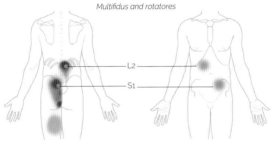

Multifidus

Action
Rotate and assist in extension of vertebral column.

Basic Functional Movement
Helps maintain good posture and spinal stability during standing, sitting, and all movements.

Referred Pain Patterns
Multifidus: localized and anteriorly to abdomen. S1 leads to coccydynia.
Rotatores: localized to medial pain.

Indications
Deep/persistent low backache, vertebral alignment problems, facilitated segment—localized paraspinal erythema, coccydynia.

Causes
Poor posture, playing musical instruments, lying on front with head propped up, poor glasses, upper crossed pattern, kyphosis, scoliosis, wear and tear, cold drafts/air conditioning, vertebral alignment issues, certain sports (e.g., archery), tight shirt/tie, depression.

Differential Diagnosis
Angina. Visceral pain. Radiculopathy. Ligamentous, discogenic, sacroiliac. Piriformis. Pathological: aortic aneurysm. Visceral pathology. Space-occupying lesion. Pelvic inflammatory disease.

Connections
Pectoralis major.

Splenius Capitis and Splenius Cervicis

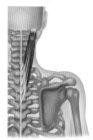
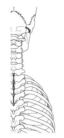

Splenius capitis

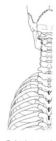
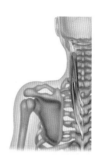

Splenius cervicis

Greek, *splenion*, bandage. **Latin**, *capitis*, of the head; *cervicis*, of the neck.

Origin
Capitis: lower part of ligamentum nuchae. Spinous processes of C7 and T1–4.
Cervicis: spinous processes of T3–6.

Insertion
Capitis: posterior aspect of mastoid process of temporal bone. Lateral part of superior nuchal line, deep to attachment of sternocleidomastoid.
Cervicis: posterior tubercles of transverse processes of C1–3.

Nerve
Capitis: dorsal rami of middle cervical nerves.
Cervicis: dorsal rami of lower cervical nerves.

Action
Acting on both sides: extend head and neck.
Acting on one side: side flexes neck; rotates head to same side as contracting muscle.

Basic Functional Movement
Examples: looking up, or turning the head to look behind.

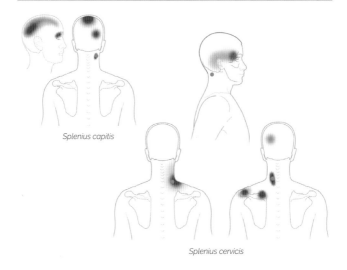

Splenius capitis

Splenius cervicis

Referred Pain Patterns
Splenius capitis: 3–5 cm zone of pain in center of vertex of skull.
Splenius cervicis: (a) upper: occipital diffuse pain, radiating via temporal region toward ipsilateral eye; (b) lower: ipsilateral pain in nape of neck.

Indications
Headache, neck pain, eye pain, blurred vision (rare), whiplash, pain from draught, postural neck pain (occupational), "internal" skull pain, neck stiffness, decreased ipsilateral rotation.

Causes
Poor posture, playing musical instruments, lying on front with head propped up, poor glasses, upper crossed pattern, kyphosis, scoliosis, wear and tear, cold drafts/air conditioning, vertebral alignment issues, certain sports (e.g., archery), tight shirt/tie, depression.

Differential Diagnosis
Other types of headache. First rib dysfunction. Torticollis. Optical problems (eyestrain). Neurological. Stress.

Connections
Trapezius, SCM, masseter, temporalis, multifidus, semispinalis capitis, suboccipital muscles, occipitofrontalis, levator scapulae, pectoralis major.

Intercostals

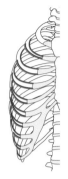

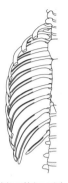

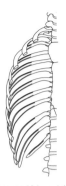

External intercostals *Internal intercostals* *Innermost intercostals*

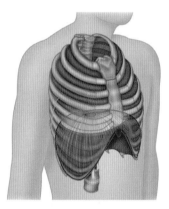

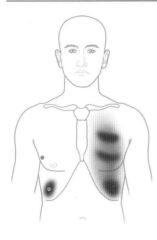

Latin, *inter*, between; *costa*, rib; *externi*, external; *interni*, internal.

There are eleven internal and external intercostals on each side of the ribcage.

Origin
External: Lower border of a rib.
Internal: Upper border of a rib and costal cartilage.

Insertion
External: Upper border of rib below (fibers run obliquely forward and downward).
Internal: Lower border of rib above (fibers run obliquely forward and upward, toward the costal cartilage).

Nerve
The corresponding intercostal nerves.

Action
Contract to stabilize ribcage during various movements of trunk. Prevent intercostal space from bulging out or sucking in during respiration.

Referred Pain Patterns
Referred to ribs, usually anterior over costochondral margins.

Indications
COPD, asthma, whiplash, rib fracture, post thoracic surgery. Hyperventilation syndrome.

Causes
COPD, asthma, whiplash, rib fracture, thoracic surgery. Difficulty breathing. Respiration. Posture. Sports (rowing, swimming).

Differential Diagnosis
CVS, Exercise-induced breathing difficulties can lead to myofascial trigger points whose symptoms can be mistaken for exercise-induced asthma. Lung pathologies such as pleurisy, cardiac issues such as myopathy. Hiatus hernia, stomach pain. Costochondritis, Tietze, Notalgia paraesthetica.

Connections
Transversus abdominis, obliques, diaphragm.

Serratus Posterior Superior

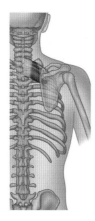

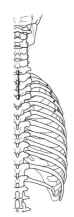

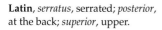

Latin, *serratus*, serrated; *posterior*, at the back; *superior*, upper.

Origin
Lower part of ligamentum nuchae. Spinous processes of C7, T1–3. Supraspinous ligaments.

Insertion
Upper borders of second to fifth ribs, lateral to their angles.

Nerve
Ventral rami of upper thoracic nerves T2–5.

Action
Raises upper ribs (probably during forced inhalation).

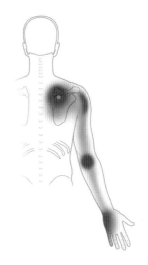

Referred Pain Patterns
Deep ache in superior region of scapula, can mimic middle trapezius but aggravated

by respiration. Pain radiates posterior shoulder and down the back of the UEX and arm, occasionally toward the ulnar border of the hand (fifth digit).

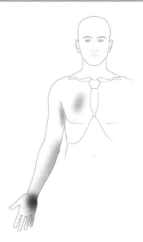

Indications
Constant deep subscapular ache, pain ipsilateral side lying, pain at rest and even when not loaded. Increased pain and difficulty on lifting outstretched arm, as scapula presses backward on the trigger points.

Causes
Occupational, musical instruments, DIY, ergonomics, pectus excavatum.

Connections
Serratus anterior, diaphragm, intercostals, levator scapulae, scalenes, pectoralis minor.

Differential Diagnosis
Scapulocostal syndrome, latissimus dorsi TPs, middle trapezius TPs, cervicogenic pain.

Serratus Posterior Inferior

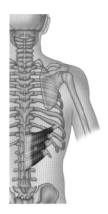

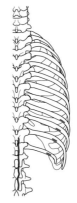

Latin, *serratus*, serrated; *posterior*, at the back; *inferior*, lower.

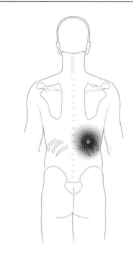

Origin
Thoracolumbar fascia, at its attachment to spinous processes of T11–12 and L1–3.

Insertion
Lower borders of last four ribs.

Nerve
Ventral rami of lower thoracic nerves T9–12.

Action
May help draw lower ribs downward and backward, resisting the pull of the diaphragm.

Referred Pain Patterns
A deep localized ache in mid back at inferolateral border ribs 8–12 and thoracolumbar junction.

Indications
Chronic mid back pain, pain on certain prolonged postures. Pain increases on movements which approximate the scapula downward toward the pelvis.

Causes
Occupational, military, computer gamers, slouching. Musical instruments like guitar. Over exertion, posture, asthma.

Differential Diagnosis
Renal, visceral, aortic aneurysm, lower bib lesion.

Connections
Iliocostalis thoracis, longissimus thoracis, quadratus lumborum, diaphragm.

Diaphragm

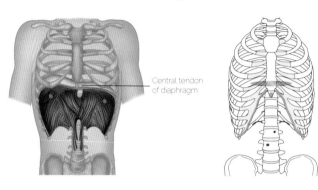

Central tendon
of diaphragm

Greek, *dia*, across; *phragma*,
partition, wall.

Thin musculotendinous structure
that separates the thoracic cavity
from the abdominal cavity.

Origin
Sternal portion: back of xiphoid
process.
Costal portion: inner surfaces of
lower six ribs and their costal
cartilages.
Lumbar portion: L1–3. Medial and
lateral arcuate ligaments.

Insertion
All fibers converge and attach
onto a central tendon, i.e., this
muscle inserts upon itself.

Nerve
Phrenic nerve (ventral rami)
C3–5.

Action
Forms floor of thoracic cavity.
Pulls central tendon downward

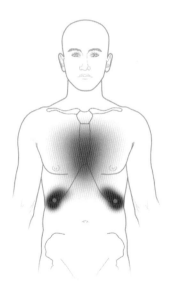

during inhalation, thereby
increasing volume of thoracic
cavity.

Basic Functional Movement

Produces about 60% of breathing capacity.

Non-respiratory functions: helps to expel vomit, faeces and urine from the body by increasing intra-abdominal pressure. Aids in childbirth. Prevents acid reflux by exerting pressure on the esophagus as it passes through the esophageal hiatus.

Indications

"Stitch" pain on running, heart/lung issues, anxiety and hyperventilation syndrome, asthma, COPD.

Causes

Asthma, pregnancy (abortion), emotional overload, disc problems in the lower back, running, occupational positions, trauma, weak abdominals, abdominal surgery, anxiety and hyperventilation syndrome, smoking, slumped postures.

Connections

Serratus anterior, intercostals, upper part rectus abdominis, arcuate ligaments, obliques.

External Oblique

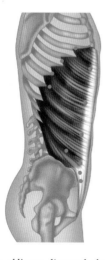 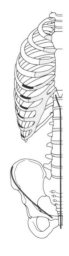

Latin, *obliquus,* diagonal, slanted; *externus,* external; *abdominis,* of the belly/stomach.

The posterior fibers of the external oblique are usually overlapped by latissimus dorsi, but in some cases there is a space

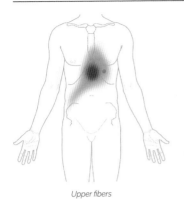

Upper fibers

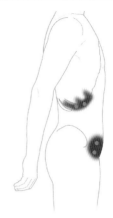

Lateral view, upper and lower fibers

between the two, known as the **lumbar triangle**, situated just above the iliac crest. The lumbar triangle is a weak point in the abdominal wall.

Origin
Muscular slips from the outer surfaces of the lower eight ribs.

Insertion
Lateral lip of iliac crest. Aponeurosis ending in linea alba.

Nerve
Ventral rami of thoracic spinal nerves T5–12.

Action
Compresses abdomen, helping to support abdominal viscera against pull of gravity. Contraction of one side alone side flexes trunk to that side and rotates it to the opposite side.

Basic Functional Movement
Example: digging with a shovel.

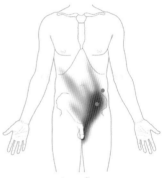

Lower fibers

Referred Pain Patterns
Viscerosomatic.
Costal margin: abdominal pain to chest.
Lower lateral: testicular pain.
Local pain.
Pubic rim: bladder pain.
Frequency/retention (urine).
Groin.

Indications

Abdominal pain and tenderness, groin pain, testicular pain, bladder pain, nausea, colic, dysmenorrhea, diarrhea, viscerosomatic pain, irritable bowel syndrome, lower crossed pattern, bedwetting in children.

Causes

Direct trauma (commonly from overexertion during sports), poor sit-up technique, prolonged cross-legged sitting, coughing, emotional stress, may be related to back pain, post-surgical (abdominal).

Differential Diagnosis

Visceral pathology including: renal, hepatic, pancreatic, diverticular disease, colitis, appendicitis, hiatus hernia, peritoneal disease—pelvic inflammatory disease, ovarian, bladder.

Connections

Transversus abdominis, internal oblique, rectus abdominis, pyramidalis.

Transversus Abdominis

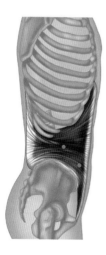 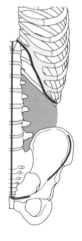

Latin, *transversus*, across, crosswise; *abdominis*, of the belly/stomach.

Origin
Anterior two-thirds of iliac crest. Lateral third of inguinal

ligament. Thoracolumbar fascia. Costal cartilages of lower six ribs.

Insertion
Aponeurosis ending in linea alba. Pubic crest and pectineal line.

Nerve
Ventral rami of thoracic spinal nerves T7–12 and L1.

Action
Compresses abdomen, helping to support abdominal viscera against pull of gravity.

Basic Functional Movement
Helps maintain good posture. Important during forced expiration, sneezing, and coughing.

Referred Pain Patterns
Costal margin: local quadrant pain, often radiating into anterior abdomen.
Suprapubic: local pain, often radiating medially and inferiorly to testes.

Indications
Groin pain, testicular pain, heartburn, nausea, vomiting, bloating, diarrhea, discogenic pain from the lumbar spine, lower crossed pattern, bedwetting in children.

Causes
Direct trauma (commonly from overexertion during sports), poor sit-up technique, prolonged

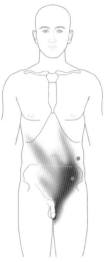

Lateral abdominals

cross-legged sitting, coughing, emotional stress, may be related to back pain, post-surgical (abdominal).

Differential Diagnosis
Visceral pathology including: renal, hepatic, pancreatic, diverticular disease, colitis, appendicitis, hiatus hernia, peritoneal disease—pelvic inflammatory disease, ovarian, bladder, testicular pathology, e.g., varicocele, nonspecific urethritis.

Connections
Obliques, rectus abdominis, pyramidalis.

Rectus Abdominis

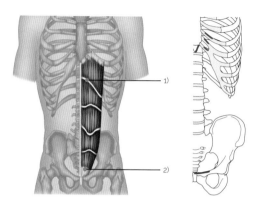

1)

2)

Latin, *rectus*, straight; *abdominis*, of the belly/stomach.

Rectus abdominis consists of tendinous bands divided into three or four bellies, each sheathed in aponeurotic fibers from the lateral abdominal muscles. These fibers converge centrally to form the linea alba. Situated anterior to the lower part of rectus abdominis is a frequently absent muscle called *pyramidalis*, which arises from the pubic crest and inserts into the linea alba. It tenses the linea alba, for reasons unknown.

Origin
Pubic crest, pubic tubercle, and symphysis pubis.

Insertion
Anterior surface of xiphoid process. Fifth, sixth, and seventh costal cartilages.

Nerve
Ventral rami of thoracic nerves T5–12.

Action
Flexes lumbar spine and pulls ribcage down. Stabilizes pelvis during walking.

Basic Functional Movement
Example: initiating getting out of a low chair.

Referred Pain Patterns
Upper fibers: horizontal mid-back pain; heartburn and indigestion.
Lower fibers: pain between pubis and umbilicus, causing dysmenorrhea.
Lateral fibers: pseudoappendicitis; McBurney's point.

Indications
Heartburn, colic, dysmenorrhea, nausea, vomiting, sense of

being full, horizontal back pain, lower crossed pattern, rib pain, testicular pain, diaphragm and breathing issues.

Causes
Direct trauma, postural, visceroptosis (commonly from overexertion during sports), poor sit-up technique, prolonged cross-legged sitting, coughing, emotional stress, may be related to back pain, post-surgical (abdominal).

Differential Diagnosis
Visceral pathology including: renal, hepatic, pancreatic, diverticular disease, colitis, appendicitis, hiatus hernia, peritoneal disease—pelvic inflammatory disease, ovarian, bladder. Appendicitis. Gynecological disease. Umbilical/incisional—hernia. Latissimus dorsi.

Connections
Transversus abdominis, obliques, pyramidalis.

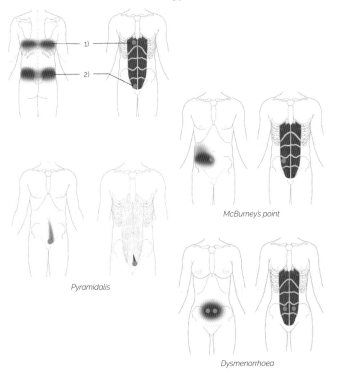

1)
2)

Pyramidalis

McBurney's point

Dysmenorrhoea

Quadratus Lumborum

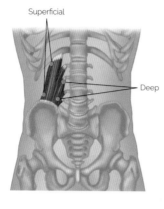
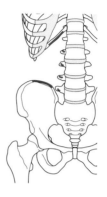

Latin, *quadratus,* squared;
lumborum, of the lower back.

Origin
Transverse process of L5.
Posterior part of iliac crest.
Iliolumbar ligament.

Insertion
Medial part of lower border of
twelfth rib. Transverse processes
of L1–4.

Nerve
Ventral rami of T12, L1–4.

Action
Side flexes vertebral column.
Fixes twelfth rib during deep
respiration (e.g., helps stabilize
diaphragm for singers exercising
voice control). Helps extend
lumbar part of vertebral column
and gives it lateral stability.

Basic Functional Movement
Example: bending sideways from
sitting to pick up an object from
the floor.

Referred Pain Patterns
Several "zones" of pain at: lower
abdomen, sacroiliac joint (upper
pole), lower buttock, upper hip,
and greater trochanter.

Indications
Renal tubular acidosis,
discogenic list scoliosis,
mechanical low back pain,
walking stick/cast for fracture,
hip and buttock pain, greater
trochanteric pain (on sleep),
pain turning in bed, pain
standing upright, persistent
deep lower backache at rest,
pain on coughing and sneezing
(Valsalva's maneuver), pain
on sexual intercourse, patient
presents with a functional list

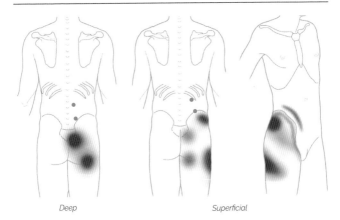

Deep   *Superficial*

to one side, may be associated with acute low back pain and radiations into leg(s), post kidney stone treatment, sciatica.

Causes

Disc problems in lower back, or facet or spinal joint issues (such as degeneration, sacroiliac joint issues, and spondylolisthesis or spondylolysis in lumbar spine), repetitive strain, gardening, putting on shoes/socks while standing, housework, occupational positions, soft mattress, trauma, weak abdominals, short leg on one side (PSLE).

Differential Diagnosis

Sacroiliitis. Bursitis of hip. Radiculopathy (lumbar). Disc pain (lumbar). Ligamentous pain (iliolumbar/lumbosacral). Spondylosis. Spondyloarthropathy. Stenosis (spinal). Spondylolisthesis. Rib dysfunction (lower).

Connections

Glutes, TFL, pyramidalis, iliopsoas, pelvic floor, sciatica, hernia, testicular/scrotal, transversus abdominis, external oblique, diaphragm.

Iliopsoas

Some of the upper fibers of psoas major may insert by a long tendon into the iliopubic eminence to form psoas minor, which has little function and is absent in about 40% of people. Bilateral contraction of psoas major will increase lumbar lordosis.

Together, psoas major and iliacus are referred to as the *iliopsoas*.

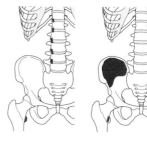

Psoas major   *Iliacus*

Nerve
Ventral rami of lumbar nerves L1–3 (psoas minor innervated from L1, 2).

Iliacus

Latin, *iliacus*, relating to the loin.

Origin
Superior two-thirds of iliac fossa. Anterior sacroiliac and iliolumbar ligaments. Upper lateral part of sacrum.

Insertion
Lesser trochanter of femur.

Nerve
Femoral nerve L2–4.

Action
Main flexors of hip joint. Flex and laterally rotate thigh, as in kicking a football. Bring leg forward in walking or running. Acting from their insertion, they flex the trunk, as in sitting up from supine position.

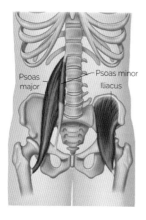

Psoas major

Greek, *psoa*, muscle of the loins. **Latin**, *major*, larger.

Origin
Transverse processes of L1–5. Bodies of T12–L5 and the intervertebral discs between each vertebra.

Insertion
Lesser trochanter of femur.

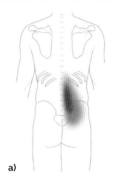

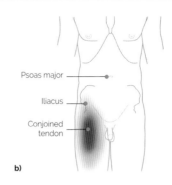

Psoas major

Iliacus

Conjoined
tendon

a)

b)

Basic Functional Movement
Examples: going up a step or walking up an incline.

Referred Pain Patterns
(a) Strong vertical ipsilateral paraspinal pain along lumbar spine, diffusely radiating laterally 3–7 cm;
(b) Strong zone of pain 5–8 cm top of anterior thigh, within diffuse zone from ASIS to upper half of thigh.

Indications
Low back pain, groin pain, increased (hyper) lordosis of lumbar spine, anterior thigh pain, pain prominent in lying to sitting up, scoliosis, asymmetry (pelvic).

Causes
Pregnancy (abortion), emotional overload, large lordosis, disc problems in lower back, or facet or spinal joint issues (such as degeneration, sacroiliac joint issues, and spondylolisthesis or spondylolysis in lumbar spine), running, repetitive strain, gardening, putting on shoes/socks while standing, housework, occupational positions, soft mattress, trauma, weak abdominals, abdominal surgery, sexual activity, short leg on one side (PSLE).

Differential Diagnosis
Osteoarthritis of hip. Appendicitis. Femoral neuropathy. Meralgia paresthetica. L4–5 disc. Bursitis. Quadriceps injury. Mechanical back dysfunction. Hernia (inguinal/femoral). Gastrointestinal. Rheumatoid arthritis. Space-occupying lesions.

Connections
Quadratus lumborum, multifidus, erector spinae, quadriceps, hip rotators, pectineus, TFL, adductors (longus/brevis), femoropatellar joint, diaphragm, rectus abdominis, obliques, pyramidalis.

Pelvic Floor Muscles

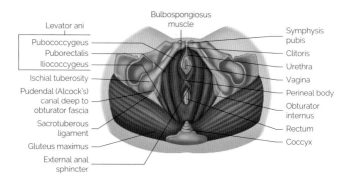

The pelvic floor is a muscular layer that spans the bottom of the pelvis and separates the pelvic cavity from the perineum below. It is made up mainly of the levator ani muscle and to a lesser extent the smaller coccygeus muscle.

The muscles that constitute the pelvic wall are **obturator internus** (page 168) and **piriformis** (page 164).

Also known as the pelvic diaphragm, the pelvic floor is a bowl-like structure that supports the pelvic viscera (urinary bladder and intestines in men, and additionally the uterus in women). Furthermore, it plays a vital role in maintaining continence as part of the urinary and anal sphincters, but also helps to produce increases in intra-abdominal pressure, to assist micturition, defecation, and childbirth.

These muscles don't have good trigger point data and are less clinically useful, but below is an interpretation of what is available.

Referred Pain Patterns
An oval shaped map centered on the coccyx and internally to gluteus maximus folds.

Indications
Lumbalgia, iliosacral pain, menstrual problems, pelvic pain, lower lumbar disc pathology. Interstitial cystitis (IC).

Causes
Pelvic inflammatory disease, postpartum, pregnancy, anal pain, and painful bowel movements, buttock pain, colic, dysmenorrhea, groin pain,

Trigger Points and Low Back Pain

Low back pain (LBP) may be multi-factorial and the presence of trigger points may be one of the factors; either maintaining, triggering, or even causative in both acute and chronic presentations.

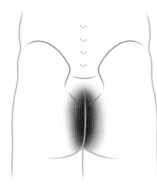

In general, the position for trigger points in the lumbo-pelvic region will depend upon what the body is trying to achieve. A thorough case history and diagnosis is therefore essential. Is the body trying to protect and defend itself? For example, if there is an acute disc, the body often lists into a protective scoliosis using the **QL** (page 90), **erector spinae/multifidus**, (pages 70/74) and **serratus posterior inferior** (page 81).

iliosacral pain, impotence due to nerve entrapments, low back pain (lumbalgia), painful intercourse (dyspareunia), sciatica, stress incontinence, or anal/genital/perineal pain.

In some cases, trigger points can cause pain similar to radiculopathic pain. For example, **Gmin** (page 163) has an extensive pain referral pattern which may mimic the L5/S1 dermatome.

Differential Diagnosis
Obturator internus issues, prolapse, hemorrhoids, coccydynia.

Connections
Coccygeus, pubococcygeus.

Conditions like sciatica may also have an origin in a taut **piriformis** (page 164). The presence of trigger points may add to the nociceptive drive to the dorsal horn, and be involved in both peripheral and central sensitization.

Common trigger point sources of back pain: **Rectus abdominis** (page 88), **erector spinae** (page 70), **multifidus** (page 74), **iliopsoas** (page 92), **Gmax** (page 158), **piriformis** (page 164), **lower fibers of latissimus dorsi** (page 111).

Pain Sitting to Standing

If your patient has pain changing positions from sitting to standing, it is well worth looking for TPs in the QL.

CHAPTER 4

Muscles of the Shoulder and Arm

Many common conditions affecting the shoulder, upper arm, and elbow can be caused entirely or in part by trigger points, including frozen shoulder, rotator cuff syndrome, and tennis elbow.

Trigger points in the subscapularis primarily cause severe, painful restricted range of motion and frozen shoulder, as in frozen shoulder syndrome. This is often not a specific diagnosis of what is occurring. As symptoms worsen, the patient is unable to lift their arm above shoulder level or reach across their chest. As trigger points from other muscles become involved, they each add their own pain patterns—typically pectoralis major, latissimus dorsi, supraspinatus, and teres major.

Rotator cuff injuries can be caused by sudden stress on muscles that are already tight from trigger point contractions, and trigger points will form after the injury and prevent proper healing. Rotator cuff syndromes make up 70% of all shoulder problems presenting to clinicians. It is well worth checking for trigger points in the triceps brachii, infraspinatus, subscapularis, and long head of biceps brachii for this issue, as well as for many other shoulder problems.

Tennis elbow (pain on the outside of the elbow) can be associated with trigger points in anconeus and biceps brachii, plus supinator, brachioradialis, extensor carpi radialis longus, and brachialis muscles (see Chapter 5).

Trapezius

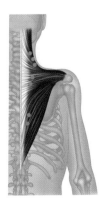 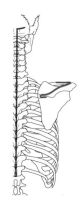

Greek, *trapezoides*, table shaped.

The left and right trapezius viewed as a whole create a trapezium in shape, thus giving this muscle its name.

Origin
Medial third of superior nuchal line of occipital bone. External occipital protuberance. Ligamentum nuchae. Spinous processes and supraspinous ligaments of C7 and T1–12.

Insertion
Superior edge of crest of spine of scapula. Medial border of acromion. Posterior border of lateral one-third of clavicle.

Nerve
Motor supply: accessory nerve (XI).

Sensory supply (proprioception): ventral rami of cervical nerves C3 and 4.

Action
Powerful elevator of the scapula; rotates the scapula during abduction of humerus above horizontal.
Middle fibers retract scapula. Lower fibers depress scapula, particularly against resistance, as when using hands to get up from a chair.

Basic Functional Movement
Example: painting a ceiling: upper and lower fibers working together.

Referred Pain Patterns
Upper fibers: pain and tenderness, posterior and lateral aspect of upper neck. Temporal region and angle of jaw.

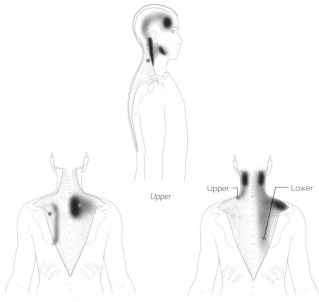

Upper

Upper — Lower

Middle

Middle fibers: local pain, radiating medially to spine.
Lower fibers: posterior cervical spine, mastoid area, area above spine of scapula.

Indications
Chronic tension and neck ache, stress headache, cervical spine pain, whiplash, tension/cluster headache, facial/jaw pain, neck pain and stiffness, upper shoulder pain, mid-back pain, dizziness, eye pain, emotional stress, depression.

Causes
Habitual postures, work, stress, neck problems, shoulder muscle weakness, telephone to ear, scoliosis, sports-related (e.g., tennis, golf), playing musical instruments.

Differential Diagnosis
Capsular-ligamentous apparatus. Articular dysfunction (facet).

Connections
Masseter, temporalis, occipitalis, levator scapulae, semispinalis, iliocostalis, clavicular part of SCM, neck/jaw/shoulder joint muscles.

Levator Scapulae

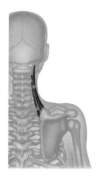
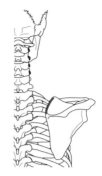

Latin, *levare*, to lift; *scapulae*, of the shoulder blade.

Levator scapulae is deep to sternocleidomastoid and trapezius.

Origin
Transverse processes of C1–2, and posterior tubercles of transverse processes of C3–4.

Insertion
Posterior surface of medial border of scapula from superior angle to root of spine of scapula.

Nerve
Ventral rami of C3 and C4 spinal nerves and dorsal scapular nerve (C5).

Action
Elevates scapula. Helps retract scapula. Helps side flex neck.

Basic Functional Movement
Example: carrying a heavy bag.

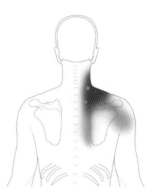

Referred Pain Patterns
Triangular pattern from top of scapula to nape of neck. Slight overspill to medial border of scapula and posterior glenohumeral joint.

Indications
Stiff and painful neck with limited rotation of cervical spine, long-term use of walking stick, neck pain and stiffness, problems turning neck (e.g., driving).

Causes

RTA, holding telephone ear to shoulder, side sleeping with wrong pillows, backpacks, poor posture, sustained habits or occupation, TV/monitor position, stress and tension, cold/flu or cold sores, sports (swimming front crawl).

Differential Diagnosis

Scapulothoracic joint dysfunction; winging of scapula. Apophysitis and capsular-ligamentous apparatus. Shoulder impingement syndromes.

Connections

Trapezius, rhomboids, splenius cervicis, erector spinae, scalenes, SCM.

Rhomboids

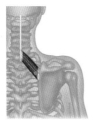

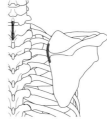

Rhomboid minor

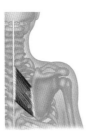

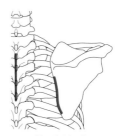

Rhomboid major

Greek, *rhomboeides*, parallelogram shaped, with only opposite sides and angles equal. **Latin**, *minor*, smaller; *major*, larger.

Rhomboid major runs parallel to, and is often continuous with, rhomboid minor. So named because of their shape.

Origin
Minor: spinous processes of C7–T1. Lower part of ligamentum nuchae.
Major: spinous processes of T2–5 and intervening supraspinous ligaments.

Insertion
Minor: posterior surface of medial border of scapula at the root of spine of scapula.
Major: posterior surface of medial border of scapula from the root of spine of scapula to the inferior angle.

Nerve
Dorsal scapular nerve C4, 5.

Action
Elevates and retracts scapula.

Basic Functional Movement
Example: pulling something toward you, such as opening a drawer.

Referred Pain Patterns
Medial border of scapula, wrapping around superior aspect of spine of scapula toward acromion process.

Indications
Localized pain/chronic aching (C7–T5) region—medial or periscapular, scapulothoracic joint grinding/grating/crunching, shoulder snapping/

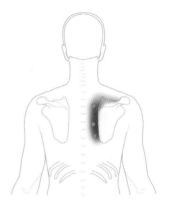

grating/clicking, aching across spinal border of shoulder blade, round shoulders, postural.

Causes
Chronic poor posture (round shouldered), shortened pectoralis minor, sports and overhead throwing, posture and habits.

Differential Diagnosis
Scapulocostal syndrome. Fibromyalgia.

Connections
Levator scapulae, middle trapezius, infraspinatus, scalenes, latissimus dorsi, serratus posterior inferior.

Serratus Anterior

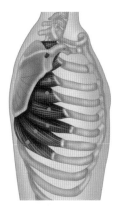 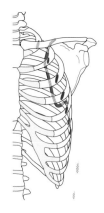

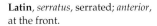

Latin, *serratus*, serrated; *anterior*, at the front.

Serratus anterior forms the medial wall of the axilla, along with the upper five ribs. It is a large muscle composed of a series of finger-like slips. The lower slips interdigitate with the origin of the external oblique.

Origin
Lateral surfaces of upper eight or nine ribs and deep fascia covering the related intercostal spaces.

Insertion
Anterior surface of medial border of scapula.

Nerve
Long thoracic nerve C5–7.

Action
Rotates scapula for abduction and flexion of arm. Protracts scapula (pulls it forward on the ribs and holds it closely into the chest wall), facilitating pushing movements, such as press-ups or punching.

Basic Functional Movement
Examples: reaching forward for something barely within reach, pushing a door open.

Referred Pain Patterns
Local: where each digitation attaches to rib.
Central: rib (6–8), localized pain, radiating anteriorly and posteriorly in a 5–10 cm patch. Pain inferior angle of scapula. Pain in ulnar aspect of upper extremity.

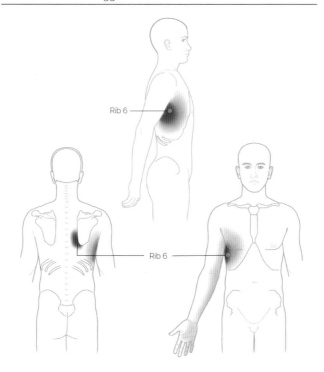

Rib 6

Rib 6

Indications
Chest pain which does not abate with rest, breast pain and sensitivity, panic attacks, dyspnea, chronic cough, asthma, renal tubular acidosis, scapula winging, chronic "stitch" on running, stress, "stitch" in the side of rib cage, pain on deep breathing, breast sensitivity, heart attack-type pain.

Causes
Severe coughing attack (maybe correlated with emphysema), overuse in sports (e.g., tennis, swimming, boxing, pull-ups and push-ups, weight lifting, gymnastics), prolonged lifting of large heavy objects, anxiety.

Differential Diagnosis
T7/T8 intercostal nerve entrapment. Herpes zoster. Local vertebral alignment. Rib lesions. Breast pathologies. Reflex-sympathetic dystrophy.

Connections
Pectoralis major, SCM, middle scalene, trapezius, rhomboids, diaphragm, external oblique.

Pectoralis Minor

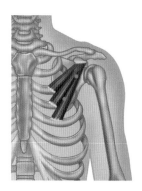
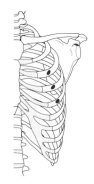

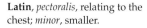

Latin, *pectoralis*, relating to the chest; *minor*, smaller.

Pectoralis minor is a flat triangular muscle lying posterior to, and concealed by, pectoralis major.

Origin
Outer surfaces of third to fifth ribs, and fascia of the corresponding intercostal spaces.

Insertion
Coracoid process of scapula.

Nerve
Medial pectoral nerve C5, (6), 7, 8, T1.

Action
Draws tip of shoulder downward. Protracts scapula. Raises ribs during forced inspiration (i.e., it is an accessory

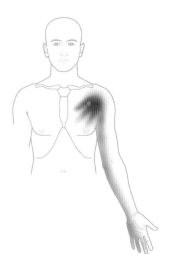

muscle of inspiration, if the scapula is stabilized by the rhomboids and trapezius).

Basic Functional Movement
Example: pushing on the arms of a chair to stand up.

Referred Pain Patterns
Chest flaring in the muscle fiber direction, often deep. Patterns radiate into medial border of entire upper extremity to medial two and a half fingers.

Indications
Upper crossed postural issues, myopathic plexopathy of axillary nerve plexus, range of shoulder problems.

Causes
Chronic poor posture (round shouldered/upper crossed patterns), shoulder-intense sports such as throwing, occupational positions, musical instruments, RTA—WAD II/III (whiplash).

Differential Diagnosis
CVS—heart-attack/MI. Ulnar neuropathy. Cubital tunnel syndrome. Short head biceps tendinopathy.

Connections
Coracobrachialis, medial biceps, short head biceps tendon, infraspinatus, rhomboids, serratus anterior.

Subclavius

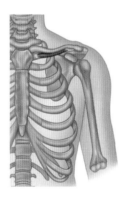
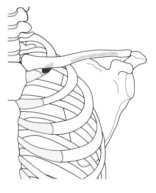

Latin, *sub*, under; *clavis*, key.

Subclavius lies deep to pectoralis major, and passes between the clavicle and first rib.

Origin
First rib at junction between rib and costal cartilage.

Insertion
Groove on inferior surface of middle one-third of clavicle.

Nerve
Nerve to subclavius C5, 6.

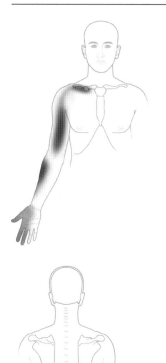

Referred Pain Patterns
Pain is referred to the ipsilateral biceps brachii and lateral forearm. Locally, pain will be experienced just below the clavicle. Pain may be felt as pins and needles in the arm, shoulder, and hand. The pain typically bypasses the elbow and wrist, and runs to the radial half of the hand, thumb, and middle finger.

Indications
Post clavicular injury, shoulder dysfunction, scoliosis.

Causes
Poor posture while sitting, round-shouldered/upper crossed pattern postures, heavy lifting, chilling of muscle in air conditioning, immobilization of shoulder or arm in cast or sling, anxiety and poor breathing, sports overload (e.g., weight training, rowing, boxing, push-ups).

Differential Diagnosis
C5–C6 radiculopathy. Biceps tendinitis. Rotator cuff muscle lesions. Intrathoracic pathology. Esophageal pathology. Tietze's syndrome. Ischemic heart disease (angina). Thoracic outlet syndrome. Median nerve dysfunction. AC joint dysfunction.

Action
Draws tip of shoulder downward. Pulls clavicle medially to stabilize sternoclavicular joint.

Connections
Coracobrachialis, pectoralis minor, serratus anterior.

Pectoralis Major

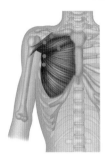

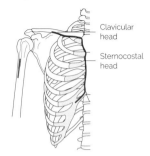

Clavicular head

Sternocostal head

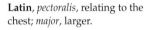

Latin, *pectoralis*, relating to the chest; *major*, larger.

Pectoralis major is one of the main climbing muscles, pulling the body up to the fixed arm.

Origin
Clavicular head: anterior surface of medial half of clavicle.
Sternocostal head: anterior surface of sternum. First seven costal cartilages. Sternal end of sixth rib. Aponeurosis of external oblique.

Insertion
Lateral lip of intertubercular sulcus of humerus.

Nerve
Medial and lateral pectoral nerves: *clavicular head*: C5, 6; *sternocostal head*: C6–8, T1.

Action
Flexion, adduction, and medial rotation of arm at glenohumeral joint.

Clavicular head: flexion of extended arm.
Sternocostal head: extension of flexed arm.

Basic Functional Movement
Clavicular head: brings the arm forward and across the body, e.g., as in applying deodorant to the opposite armpit.
Sternocostal head: pulling something down from above, e.g., a rope in bell-ringing.

Referred Pain Patterns
Clavicular head: local pain, radiating to anterior deltoid and long head of biceps brachii area.
Sternal head: "acute" back pain into anterior chest wall in a 10–20 cm patch of diffuse pain around medial border of upper extremity. Stronger pain below medial epicondyle in a 5 cm patch, diffuse pain into fourth and fifth digits.
Costal portion: fifth and sixth ribs leads to severe cardiac referral (even at night). Intense breast

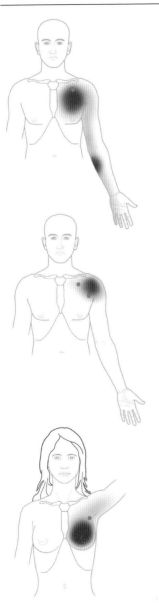

pain (10–15 cm patch). Diffuse radiations into axillary tail, and into axilla.

Indications
Post myocardial infarct rehabilitation, cardiac arrhythmia, mid-scapular back pain, breast pain and hypersensitivity, thoracic outlet syndrome, anterior shoulder pain, golfer's and tennis elbow, round-shouldered postures, chest pain, chronic fatigue, hyperventilation syndrome.

Causes
Poor posture while sitting, round-shouldered postures, heavy lifting, chilling of muscle in air conditioning, immobilization of shoulder or arm in cast or sling, anxiety and poor breathing, sports overload (e.g., weight training, rowing, boxing, push-ups).

Differential Diagnosis
C5–C6 radiculopathy. Biceps tendinitis. Rotator cuff muscle lesions. Intrathoracic pathology. Esophageal pathology. Tietze's syndrome. Ischemic heart disease (angina). Thoracic outlet syndrome.

Connections
Latissimus dorsi, subscapularis, teres minor, infraspinatus, trapezius (middle fibers), serratus anterior, scalenes, deltoid, coracobrachialis, sternalis, SCM, paraspinals.

Sternalis

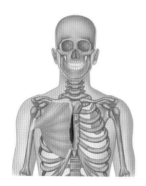 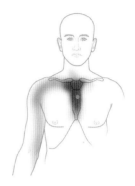

Latin, *sternalis*, relating to the sternum.

Present in only 7–8% of people, trigger points in this muscle can be a serious source of chronic pain for some.

Origin
Mostly located superficially and perpendicular to pectoralis major, and on one or both sides of sternum.

Insertion
Variable insertion—pectoral fascia, lower ribs, costal cartilage, and/or rectus abdominis/external oblique sheath (aponeurosis).

Nerve
External/internal thoracic, pectoral, and/or intercostal nerves.

Action
Works with pectoralis major, bracing the sternum.

Basic Functional Movement
May function as a proprioceptive sensor for thoracic wall movements, take part in movement of shoulder joint, or have additional role in elevation of chest wall.

Referred Pain Patterns
Across sternum, either unilaterally or bilaterally, radiating into chest wall and inner biceps region.

Indications
Chest asymmetry, chest pain.

Causes
Whiplash (seatbelt), cardiothoracic surgery, mastectomy, breast augmentation, exercise induced.

Differential Diagnosis
TseTse.

Connections
Clavipectoral fascia, lower ribs, costal cartilages, rectus sheath, aponeurosis of external oblique.

Latissimus Dorsi

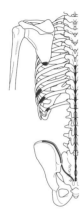 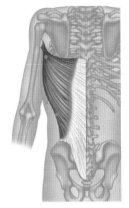

Latin, *latissimus*, widest; *dorsi*, of the back.

Origin
Spinous processes of lower six thoracic vertebrae and related interspinous ligaments; via thoracolumbar fascia (a broad sheet of tendon) to the spinous processes of lumbar vertebrae, related interspinous ligaments, and iliac crest. Lower three or four ribs.

Insertion
Twists to insert into the floor of intertubercular sulcus of humerus, just below the shoulder joint.

Nerve
Thoracodorsal nerve C6–8.

Action
Adduction, medial rotation, and extension of the arm at the glenohumeral joint. It is one of the chief climbing muscles, since it pulls shoulders downward and backward, and pulls trunk up to the fixed arms (therefore also active in crawl swimming stroke). Assists in forced inspiration, by raising lower ribs.

Basic Functional Movement
Example: pushing on the arms of a chair to stand up.

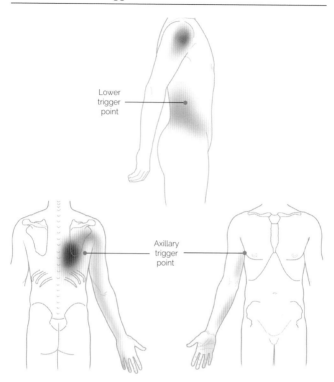

Lower trigger point

Axillary trigger point

Referred Pain Patterns

Axillary trigger point: a 5–10 cm zone of pain at inferior angle of scapula, with diffuse pain radiating into medial upper extremity into ulnar aspect of hand.

Lower lateral trigger point: triangular pattern from trigger point into brim of pelvis and regimental badge area.

Indications

"Thoracic" back pain that is constant in nature and unrelated to activity, frozen shoulder, thoracic outlet syndrome, back pain turning in bed, dull ache under shoulder blade, sharp pain in back of shoulder when resting on elbows, pain when reaching up to a shelf or changing a light bulb.

Causes

Golf, racquet sports, swimming, baseball, cricket, rowing, heavy lifting, gym related, gardening, poor-fitting bra.

Differential Diagnosis
C7 neuropathy. Ulnar neuropathy. Subscapular nerve entrapment. Axillary neuropathy. Thoracic outlet syndrome. Cardiopulmonary diseases.

Connections
Rhomboids, trapezius (middle fibers), teres major, scalenes, subscapularis, iliocostalis, serratus anterior, serratus posterior inferior.

Deltoid

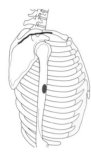

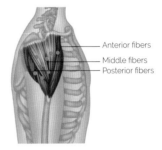

Anterior fibers
Middle fibers
Posterior fibers

Greek, *deltoeides*, shaped like the Greek capital letter delta (Δ).

Deltoid is composed of three parts: anterior, middle, and posterior. Only the middle part is multipennate, probably because its mechanical disadvantage of abduction of the shoulder joint requires extra strength.

Origin
Anterior fibers: anterior border of lateral one-third of clavicle.
Middle fibers: lateral margin of acromion process.
Posterior fibers: inferior edge of crest of spine of scapula.

Insertion
Deltoid tuberosity of humerus.

Nerve
Axillary nerve C5, 6.

Action
Major abductor of the arm (abducts arm beyond initial 15 degrees, which is done by supraspinatus); anterior fibers assist in flexing the arm; posterior fibers assist in extending the arm.

Basic Functional Movement
Examples: reaching for something out to the side, raising the arm to wave.

Referred Pain Patterns
Generally localized to trigger point and within a 5–10 cm zone.

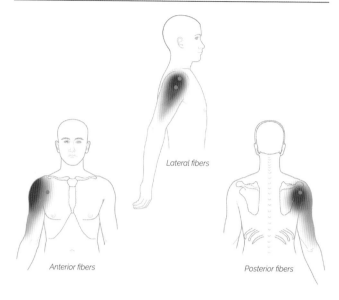

Lateral fibers

Anterior fibers

Posterior fibers

Indications

Post-trauma rehabilitation, shoulder pain, decreased ROM (esp. in abduction), shoulder pain which worsens with motion and eases at rest, reduced ROM and some loss of strength above 90 degrees.

Causes

Swimming, weight lifting, soccer (blows), basketball, jerky and vigorous repetitive movements, fishing, power tools, sudden blows, rifle rebound, skiing falls, injections into shoulder, dislocations, holding small baby.

Differential Diagnosis

Impingement syndromes. Sub-acromial bursitis. C5 radiculopathy. Rotator cuff tendinopathy. Osteoarthritis of glenohumeral or acromioclavicular joint.

Connections

Supraspinatus, infraspinatus, biceps brachii, teres minor, subscapularis, pectoralis major (clavicular head), rotator cuff issues, tendinitis, arthritis, C5 nerve issues, neck problems, often satellite trigger points from other problems (e.g., scalenes, pectoralis major), long head biceps brachii tendon problems.

Supraspinatus

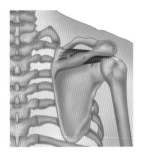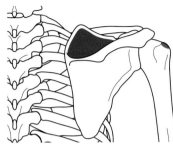

Latin, *supra*, above; *spina*, spine.

Supraspinatus is a member of the rotator cuff, which also includes teres minor, infraspinatus, and subscapularis.

Origin
Medial two-thirds of supraspinous fossa of scapula and deep fascia that covers the muscle.

Insertion
Most superior facet on the greater tubercle of humerus.

Nerve
Suprascapular nerve C5, 6.

Action
Initiates abduction of arm to 15 degrees at glenohumeral joint (at which point deltoid takes over).

Basic Functional Movement
Example: holding a shopping bag away from the side of the body.

Referred Pain Patterns
Belly: deep ache in regimental badge area (4–6 cm). Ellipse leads to zone of pain in lateral epicondyle/radial head. Diffuse pain into lateral forearm. *Insertion:* localized zone of pain 5–8 cm over deltoid.

Indications
Loss of power in abduction, painful arc syndrome, night pain/ache, subacromial bursitis, rotator cuff tendinopathy, deep aching in shoulder which can extend to elbow (i.e., tennis elbow) and occasionally to thumb side of wrist, can be confused with De Quervain's tenosynovitis, pain on initiation of lifting shoulder sideways, inability to reach behind back, moderately restricted range of shoulder motion, clicking/snapping sounds in shoulder joint.

Causes
Carrying heavy objects (e.g., bags, laptops, suitcases) over long distances, heavy lifting from floor to trunk of car, carrying with arms above head, sleeping

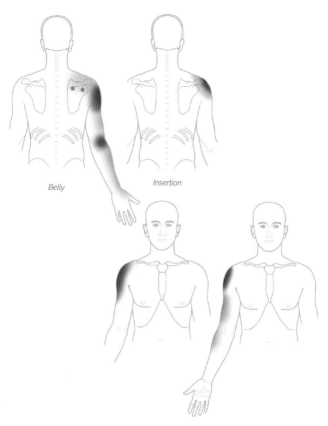

Belly

Insertion

positions with arms above head, dogs pulling on leash, falls on outstretched arm (e.g., skiing), washing/combing hair, moving heavy furniture, repetitive strain injury (RSI), prolonged computer keyboard use.

Differential Diagnosis

Phase 1 capsulitis. C5–6 radiculopathy. Subacromial bursitis (adhesive). Calcific tendinitis. Calcium boils. Rotator cuff tendinopathy.

Connections

Subscapularis, infraspinatus, deltoid, trapezius, latissimus dorsi, rotator cuff issues, biceps tendinitis.

Infraspinatus

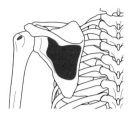

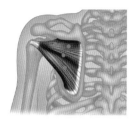

Latin, *infra*, below; *spina*, spine.

Infraspinatus is a member of the rotator cuff, which also includes supraspinatus, teres minor, and subscapularis.

Origin
Medial two-thirds of infraspinous fossa of scapula and deep fascia that covers the muscle.

Insertion
Middle facet on posterior surface of greater tubercle of humerus.

Nerve
Suprascapular nerve C5, 6.

Action
Lateral rotation of arm at glenohumeral joint.

Basic Functional Movement
Example: brushing back hair.

Referred Pain Patterns
Middle/upper cervical spine: deep anterior shoulder joint zone of 3–4 cm in region of long head

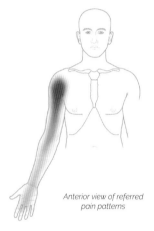

Anterior view of referred pain patterns

of biceps brachii, radiating into biceps belly then into forearm—diffuse symptoms in median nerve distribution.
Medial/scapula: to medial border of scapula.

Indications
Decreased ROM in Apley scratch test (behind back), hemiplegia, rotator cuff tendinopathy, frozen shoulder syndrome, pain in back

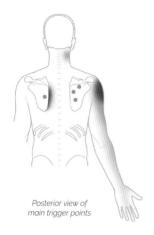

Posterior view of main trigger points

Causes
Overuse activities with arm unsupported (e.g., computer mouse, driving, tennis, weight training, water sports, ski poles), pulling objects behind body, sudden trauma from fall on outstretched arm/catching yourself when trying to stop a fall, prolonged holding of heavy objects.

Differential Diagnosis
Biceps tendinitis. C5–C6 neuropathy. Suprascapular nerve dysfunction.

and front of shoulder, night-time shoulder pain when sleeping on same/opposite side, dead-arm sensations, pain undoing bra, shoulder girdle fatigue, weakness of grip, loss of arm strength, changes in sweating (usually increased), "mouse arm" from computer mouse overuse.

Connections
Infraspinatus, subscapularis, levator scapulae, pectorals, biceps brachii (long head), anterior deltoid, teres major, latissimus dorsi, rotator cuff issues, biceps tendinitis.

Teres Minor

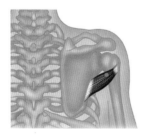

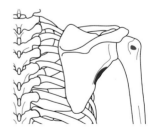

Latin, *teres*, rounded, finely shaped; *minor*, smaller.

Teres minor is a member of the rotator cuff, which also includes supraspinatus, infraspinatus, and subscapularis.

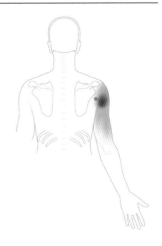

Origin
Upper two-thirds of a strip of bone on posterior surface of scapula immediately adjacent to lateral border of scapula.

Insertion
Inferior facet on greater tubercle of humerus.

Nerve
Axillary nerve C5, 6.

Action
Lateral rotation of arm at glenohumeral joint.

Basic Functional Movement
Example: brushing back hair.

Referred Pain Patterns
Localized zone (2–5 cm) of intense pain in regimental badge area, with a more diffuse elliptical zone of pain spreading in posterolateral upper extremity (above elbow).

Indications
Shoulder pain (esp. posterior), frozen shoulder syndrome, rotator cuff rehabilitation, subacromial bursitis, biceps tendinitis, shoulder pain at top outer section of shoulder blade near posterior deltoid, often associated with other shoulder problems (esp. rotator cuff issues), numbness/tingling in 4th and 5th fingers.

Causes
Reaching above 90 degrees and/or reaching behind back, gripping steering wheel in RTA, holding heavy object for long time, computer/mouse overuse syndromes.

Differential Diagnosis
C8–T1 radiculopathy. Rotator cuff tendinopathy. Shoulder–wrist–hand syndrome. Subacromial/deltoid bursitis. Shoulder impingement syndromes (painful arc). Acromioclavicular joint dysfunction.

Connections
Infraspinatus.

Subscapularis

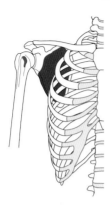 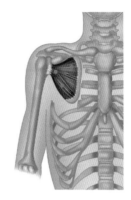

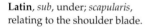

Latin, *sub*, under; *scapularis*, relating to the shoulder blade.

Subscapularis is a member of the rotator cuff, which also includes supraspinatus, infraspinatus, and teres minor.

Subscapularis constitutes the greater part of the posterior wall of the axilla.

Origin
Medial two-thirds of subscapular fossa.

Insertion
Lesser tubercle of humerus.

Nerve
Upper and lower subscapular nerves C5, 6, (7).

Action
Medial rotation of arm at glenohumeral joint.

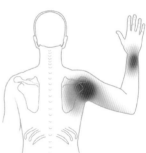

Posterior view of referred pain patterns

Basic Functional Movement
Example: reaching into the back pocket.

Referred Pain Patterns
Axillary trigger point: strong zone (5–8 cm) of pain in posterior glenohumeral joint, with a peripheral diffuse zone. Also radiating down posterior aspect of arm and anteroposterior carpals of wrist.

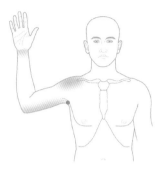

Causes

Sports-related (esp. swimming crawl, repeated forceful overhead lifting, baseball pitching/catching, cricket), post shoulder fracture/dislocation, frozen shoulder syndrome, sudden unexpected loading of shoulder (e.g., fall), post-fracture, prolonged immobility (sling).

Differential Diagnosis

Impingement syndromes.
Rotator cuff dysfunctions.
Thoracic outlet syndromes.
Cervical radiculopathy (C7).
Cardiopulmonary pathology.

Indications

Rotator cuff tendinopathy, adhesive capsulitis (frozen shoulder), decreased external rotation with abduction, severe pain over back of shoulder, restricted range of shoulder movement, inability to reach behind back, pain on throwing, clicking/popping shoulders, stroke (hemiplegia).

Connections

Infraspinatus, pectorals, teres minor, latissimus dorsi, triceps brachii, posterior deltoid, supraspinatus.

Teres Major

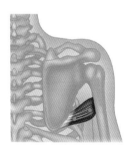

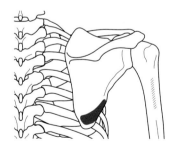

Latin, *teres*, rounded, finely shaped; *major*, larger.

Origin
Oval area on lower third of posterior surface of inferior angle of scapula.

Insertion
Medial lip of intertubercular sulcus on anterior surface of humerus.

Nerve
Lower subscapular nerve C5–7.

Action
Medial rotation and extension of arm at glenohumeral joint.

Basic Functional Movement
Example: reaching into the back pocket.

Referred Pain Patterns
Deep pain into posterior glenohumeral joint and an oval zone (5–10 cm) of pain in posterior deltoid area (can radiate strongly to long head of biceps brachii). Diffuse pain into dorsum of forearm.

Indications
Frozen shoulder syndrome, pain on reaching above head, slight pain on rest, pain when driving, impingement syndromes, sometimes misdiagnosed as thoracic outlet syndrome.

Causes
Sports-related—forceful overhead lifting, post shoulder fracture/dislocation, rotator cuff tendinopathy, sudden unexpected loading of shoulder

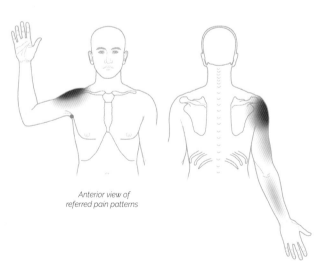

Anterior view of referred pain patterns

(e.g., fall), post-fracture, prolonged immobility (sling).

Differential Diagnosis
Impingement syndromes. Rotator cuff tendinopathy. Cervical neuropatterns (C6–C7). Thoracic outlet syndrome. Supraspinatus calcification.

Connections
Rhomboids, triceps brachii (long head), latissimus dorsi, teres minor, pectorals, posterior deltoid, C6 or C7 neck disc issue, subdeltoid bursitis.

Biceps Brachii

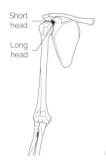
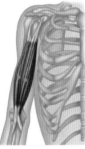
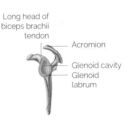

Latin, *biceps*, two-headed; *brachii*, of the arm.

Biceps brachii operates over three joints. It has two tendinous heads at its origin and two tendinous insertions. The short head forms part of the lateral wall of the axilla, along with coracobrachialis and the humerus.

Origin
Long head: supraglenoid tubercle of scapula.
Short head: tip of coracoid process.

Insertion
Radial tuberosity.

Nerve
Musculocutaneous nerve C5, 6.

Action
Powerful flexor of forearm at elbow joint. Supinates forearm. (It has been described as the muscle that puts in the corkscrew and pulls out the cork). Accessory flexor of arm at glenohumeral joint.

Basic Functional Movement
Examples: picking up an object, bringing food to the mouth.

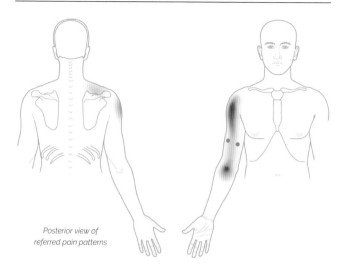

Posterior view of referred pain patterns

Referred Pain Patterns
Localized pain with intense ellipse superficially located over long head tendon. Referred pain into anterior cubital fossa.

Indications
Anterior shoulder pain with decreased arm extension, biceps tendinitis, reduced extension of arms, reduced Apley scratch test maneuver, frozen shoulder syndrome, aching pain over front of shoulder, weakness in turning palm face upward, shoulder aching.

Causes
Repetitive motion injury, throwing/sports induced (e.g., basketball, tennis), repeated actions with arm, lifting heavy objects with palm upward (e.g., weight training), musical instrument playing (e.g., violin, guitar).

Differential Diagnosis
Glenohumeral osteoarthritis. Acromioclavicular osteoarthritis. Subscapularis. Infraspinatus. Subacromial bursitis. Biceps tendinitis. C5 radiculopathy.

Connections
Subscapularis, infraspinatus, brachialis, supinator, upper trapezius, coracobrachialis, triceps brachii, anterior deltoid.

Brachialis

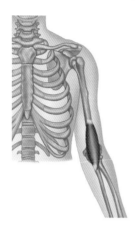
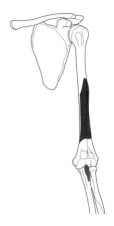

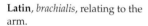

Latin, *brachialis*, relating to the arm.

Brachialis lies posterior to biceps brachii and is the main flexor of the elbow joint. Some fibers may be partly fused with brachioradialis.

Origin
Anterior aspect of humerus (medial and lateral surfaces) and adjacent intermuscular septae.

Insertion
Tuberosity of ulna.

Nerve
Musculocutaneous nerve C5, 6. Small contribution by radial nerve (C7) to lateral part of muscle.

Action
Powerful flexor of forearm at elbow joint.

Basic Functional Movement
Example: bringing food to the mouth.

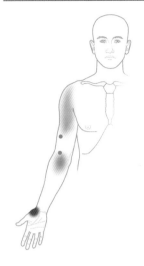
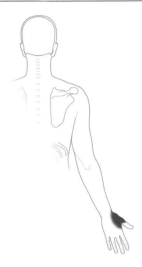

Referred Pain Patterns
Pain is felt mainly at the base of the thumb, anterior deltoid, and just below the elbow joint line. Patients often complain of tingling or numbness in the thumb and hand.

Indications
Often gets involved with SHB and other biceps problems. Thumb pain.

Causes
Overuse injuries, upper crossed postures, overhead occupation, sports, e.g., tennis or swimming. Sudden heavy lifting (biceps). Gym.

Differential Diagnosis
Carpal tunnel syndrome. De Quervain's tenosynovitis. O/A thumb joint.

Connections
Biceps brachii, coracobrachialis.

Coracobrachialis

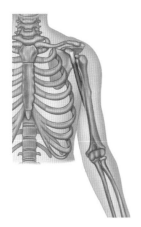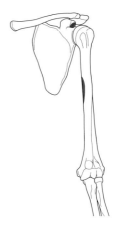

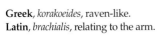

Greek, *korakoeides*, raven-like.
Latin, *brachialis*, relating to the arm.

Coracobrachialis, although acting upon the shoulder joint, is also included here because of its proximity to the other muscles of this group. Along with the short head of biceps brachii and the humerus, coracobrachialis forms the lateral wall of the axilla. Coracobrachialis is so named because it resembles a raven's beak.

Origin
Tip of coracoid process.

Insertion
Medial aspect of humerus at mid-shaft.

Nerve
Musculocutaneous nerve C5–7.

Action
Flexor of arm at glenohumeral joint.

Basic Functional Movement
Example: mopping the floor.

Referred Pain Patterns
Regimental badge, deltoid zone, posterior arm to dorsum of hand and posterior digit 3.

Indications
Overuse injuries, upper crossed syndrome, overhead occupation, sports, e.g., tennis and swimming, weight lifting.

Causes
Sudden eccentric loading. Occupational, sports.

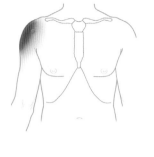

Differential Diagnosis
Infraspinatus TPs, C7 nerve root pathology, regimental badge zone pathologies, subacromial pain syndrome.

Connections
Triceps brachii, anterior deltoid.

Triceps Brachii

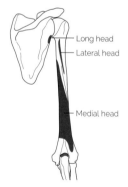

Long head
Lateral head
Medial head

Latin, *triceps*, three-headed; *brachii*, of the arm.

Triceps brachii originates from three heads which converge to form a large tendon. It is the only muscle on the back of the arm. The medial head is largely covered by the lateral and long heads.

Origin

Long head: infraglenoid tubercle of scapula.
Medial head: Posterior surface of humerus (below and medial to radial groove).
Lateral head: Posterior surface of humerus (above and lateral to radial groove).

Insertion

Posterior part of olecranon process of ulna.

Nerve

Radial nerve C6–8.

Action

Extends forearm at elbow joint. Long head can also extend and adduct arm at shoulder joint.

Basic Functional Movement

Examples: throwing objects, pushing a door shut.

Referred Pain Patterns

Long head: pain at superolateral border of shoulder, radiating diffusely down posterior upper extremity with strong zone of pain around olecranon process, and then vaguely into posterior forearm.
Medial head: 5 cm patch of pain in medial epicondyle, radiating along medial border of forearm to fourth and fifth digits.
Lateral head: strong midline pain into upper extremity, radiating vaguely into posterior forearm.

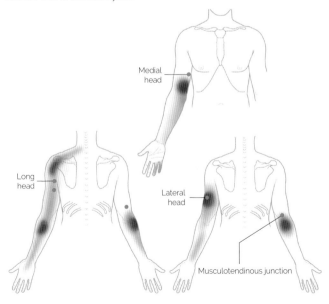

Medial head

Long head

Lateral head

Musculotendinous junction

Indications
Golfer's/tennis elbow, arthritis of elbow/shoulder, chronic use of crutches/walking stick, repetitive mechanical activities of arms, racquet sports, aching pain over front of shoulder, weakness in turning palm face upward, shoulder aching.

Causes
Repetitive motion injury, throwing/sports induced (e.g., basketball, tennis), repeated actions with arm, lifting heavy objects with palm upward (e.g., triceps-focused weight training), musical instrument playing (e.g., violin, drums, guitar).

Differential Diagnosis
Radial nerve injury. Ulnar neuropathy. C7 neuropathy (cervical disc).

Connections
Teres minor/major, latissimus dorsi, anconeus, supinator, brachioradialis, extensor carpi radialis longus, anterior deltoid.

Anconeus

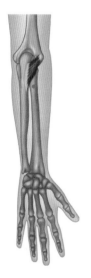
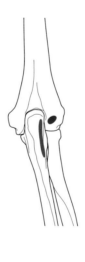
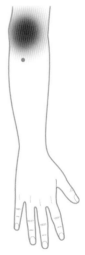

Greek, *agkon*, elbow.

Origin
Lateral epicondyle of humerus.

Insertion
Lateral surface of olecranon process and proximal posterior surface of ulna.

Nerve
Radial nerve C6, 7, 8.

Action
Abduction of ulna in pronation. Accessory extensor of elbow joint.

Basic Functional Movement
Example: pushing objects at arm's length.

Referred Pain Patterns
Localized posterior elbow pain. Often mistaken for tennis elbow. Pain experienced when trying to flex the elbow joint and supinate the forearm.

Indications
Golfer's/tennis elbow, arthritis of elbow/shoulder, chronic use of crutches/walking stick, repetitive mechanical activities of arms, racquet sports, weakness in turning palm face upward.

Causes
Repetitive motion injury, throwing/ sports induced (e.g., basketball, tennis), repeated actions with arm, lifting heavy objects with palm upward (e.g., triceps-focused weight training), musical instrument playing (e.g., violin, drums, guitar). Overuse, occupation, and RSI.

Differential Diagnosis
Radial nerve injury. Ulnar neuropathy. Triceps dysfunction. Cervical neuropathy (cervical disc).

Connections
Fibers of triceps, supinator, wrist flexors.

Trigger Points and Frozen Shoulder Syndrome (Adhesive Capsulitis)

Shoulder pain affects 60% of the population at some point and its incidence increases with age. While the most common clinical problem is rotator cuff tendinopathy (70%), then subacromial pain (10%), frozen shoulder syndrome (adhesive capsulitis [AC]), affects 3–5% of the population.

AC lasts for an average of 30 months, is more common in women 60:40, and is up to 10 times more common in diabetics. It's impact in terms of disability on quality of life is severe, esp. in the early phase (freezing) which is characterized by severe night pain, catching spasms, and reduced range of motion of 50% in all directions.

While it represents a small sub-group of shoulder pain, the way it manifests is a blue print for all shoulder problems. The body seems to shut down around the glenohumeral joint in a "default holding pattern" maintained by the **biceps** and **subscapularis** muscles. Because these muscles are always "switched on," there are secondary reflex changes such as reciprocal inhibition in the antagonists and synergists, and the nervous system is forced to recruit other muscles to do the "wrong jobs," leading to secondary trigger points. See "The Niel-Asher Technique" (NAT).

Hemiplegia—Default Posture (Cyriax Decerbration)

Orthopedic Intervention

By unlocking the secrets of AC, we are afforded an insight into the way the shoulder and other peripheral joints operate. Trigger points develop in the **biceps brachii** (page 123), **subscapularis** (page 120), and **infraspinatus** (page 117) muscles.

Furthermore, because of the chronic duration of symptoms, AC ignites central sensitization and possible autonomic nervous system involvement.

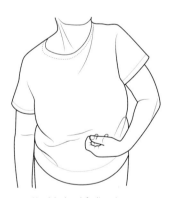

Hemiplegia—default posture "Cyriax decerbration"

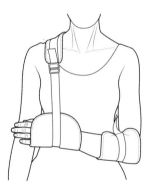

Orthopedic intervention

CHAPTER 5

Muscles of the Forearm and Hand

In everyday life, the use of computers, cell phones, gaming consoles, and other related repetitive activities has caused a huge increase in the number of patients with referred pain from trigger points in the forearm and wrist. Carpal tunnel syndrome is often incorrectly diagnosed, with trigger point symptoms from pronator teres and/or palmaris longus equally as likely. Many people misdiagnosed with carpal tunnel syndrome undergo needless surgery, while others with numbness and tingling in the fingers may be misdiagnosed with thoracic outlet syndrome. True carpal tunnel syndrome is more likely caused by using vibrating tools or by prior injuries, such as a broken or sprained wrist that caused swelling.

People are often given a brace and supports, which may afford some relief, but do little to solve problems caused by trigger points. Not only can trigger points refer pain that mimics these syndromes but the muscle tension created by these trigger points may compress nerves and even plexuses as they travel through the neck, shoulder, and forearm (myogenic compression).

More than ten muscles can be associated with wrist pain, numbness in the hand, or tingling in the fingers. In particular, check for trigger points in the scalenes, pectoralis minor, biceps brachii, brachialis, coracobrachialis, brachioradialis, wrist extensors, and wrist flexors.

Pronator Teres

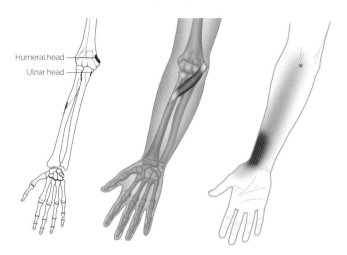

Humeral head
Ulnar head

Latin, *pronare*, to bend forward; *teres*, rounded, finely shaped.

Origin
Humeral head: medial epicondyle and adjacent supra-epicondylar ridge.
Ulnar head: medial border of coronoid process.

Insertion
Mid-lateral surface of radius (pronator tuberosity).

Nerve
Median nerve C6, 7.

Action
Pronates forearm.

Basic Functional Movement
Examples: pouring liquid from a container, turning a doorknob.

Referred Pain Patterns
Strong pain "deep" into palmar region of wrist (lateral), radiating up anterolateral forearm.

Indications
Pain in wrist (lateral), pain on supination, hairdressers (overuse of scissors), inability to "cup" hands together (esp. "cupping" and extension of wrist), shoulder pain (compensatory), wrist pain on driving.

Causes
Prolonged gripping, massaging, wrist fractures or falls, casts,

sports (e.g., forehand spin with racquet, using ski poles), occupational.

Differential Diagnosis
De Quervain's tenosynovitis. Carpal tunnel swelling. Osteoarthritis of proximal thumb joint. Distal radioulnar discopathy. Epicondylitis.

Connections
Finger flexors, scalenes, pectoralis major, pronator quadratus.

Palmaris Longus

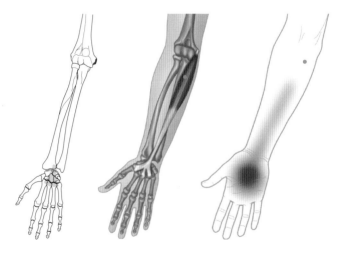

Latin, *palmaris*, relating to the palm; *longus*, long.

Absent in 14% of the population.

Origin
Medial epicondyle of humerus.

Insertion
Palmar aponeurosis of hand.

Nerve
Median nerve C(6), 7, 8.

Action
Flexes wrist joint. Tenses palmar fascia.

Basic Functional Movement
Examples: grasping a small ball, cupping the palm to drink from the hand.

Referred Pain Patterns
Diffuse pain in anterior forearm; intense pain zone 2–3 cm in

palm of hand, surrounded by a superficial zone of prickling and needle-like sensations.

Indications
Pain and "soreness" in palm of hand, tenderness in hand/palm, functional loss of power in grip, tennis elbow.

Causes
Direct trauma (e.g., fall on outstretched arm), occupational, racquet sports, digging in palm.

Differential Diagnosis
Neurogenic pain. Dupuytren's contracture. Carpal tunnel syndrome. Complex regional pain syndrome (reflex-sympathetic dystrophy). Scleroderma. Dermatomyositis.

Connections
Flexor carpi radialis, brachialis, pronator teres, wrist joints (carpals), often associated with middle head of triceps brachii.

Wrist Flexors

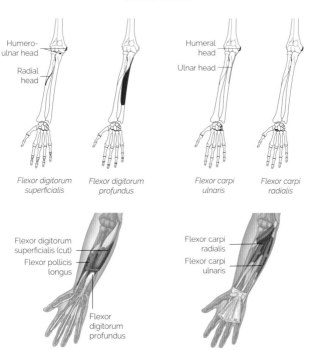

Humero-ulnar head
Radial head

Flexor digitorum superficialis

Flexor digitorum profundus

Humeral head
Ulnar head

Flexor carpi ulnaris

Flexor carpi radialis

Flexor digitorum superficialis (cut)
Flexor pollicis longus

Flexor digitorum profundus

Flexor carpi radialis
Flexor carpi ulnaris

Latin, *flectere*, to bend; *carpi*, of the wrist; *radius*, staff, spoke of wheel; *ulnaris*, of the elbow/arm; *digitus*, finger; *superficialis*, on the surface; *profundus*, deep.

Comprising: flexor carpi radialis, flexor carpi ulnaris, flexor digitorum superficialis, and flexor digitorum profundus.

Origin
Common flexor origin on anterior aspect of medial epicondyle of humerus (i.e., lower medial end of humerus).

Insertion
Carpals, metacarpals, and phalanges.

Nerve
Median nerve, C6, 7, 8, T1.

Action
Flexes wrist joint. (Flexor carpi radialis also abducts wrist joint; flexor carpi ulnaris also adducts wrist joint).

Basic Functional Movement
Examples: pulling a rope in toward you; wielding an axe or hammer; pouring liquid from a bottle; turning a door handle.

Referred Pain Patterns
Individual muscles refer to lower arm, wrist, hand, and fingers.

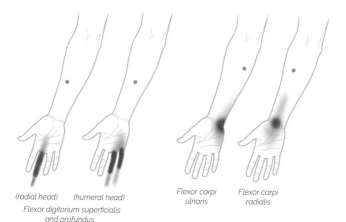

(radial head)   (humeral head)
Flexor digitorium superficialis and profundus

Flexor carpi
ulnaris

Flexor carpi
radialis

Indications
Hand/wrist/finger pain, trigger finger, cutting with scissors, gripping, golfer's elbow, RSI, hairdressers, turning hand to cupping action, tense finger flexors.

Causes
Prolonged gripping, massaging, wrist fractures or falls, casts, sports (e.g., forehand spin with racquet, using ski poles), occupational, trigger finger (flexor digitorum).

Differential Diagnosis
Ulnar neuritis. Cervical neuropathies. Carpal bone dysfunctions. De Quervain's tenosynovitis. RSI. Osteo- and rheumatoid arthritis. Radioulnar disc (distal) problems. Carpal tunnel syndrome. Medial epicondylitis.

Connections
Shoulder/upper arm muscles, scalenes, flexor pollicis longus.

Pronator Quadratus

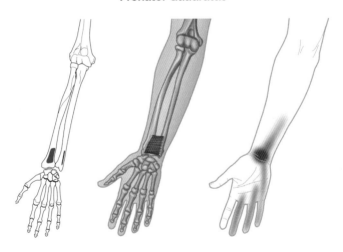

Latin, *pronare,* to bend forward; *quadratus,* squared.

Origin
Linear ridge on distal anterior surface of ulna.

Insertion
Distal anterior surface of radius.

Nerve
Anterior interosseous branch of median nerve C7, 8.

Action
Pronates forearm and hand. Helps hold radius and ulna together, reducing stress on inferior radioulnar joint.

Basic Functional Movement
Example: turning the hand downward, as in pouring a substance out of the hand.

Referred Pain Patterns
Two main pain patterns are observed. The most common pattern involves pain spreading both distally and proximally along the medial aspect of the forearm. In some cases, the pain area extends to the medial epicondyle proximally and the fifth digit distally. The second main pattern is pain spreading distally into the third and/or fourth digit.

Indications
Palmar wrist pain, pain in the articular disc.

Causes
Post wrist fracture, RSI/overuse, prolonged mouse use, racquet sports, poor stretching, playing musical instruments.

Differential Diagnosis
De Quervain's tenosynovitis, carpal tunnel syndrome, cervicopathy, disc or osseous degeneration lower cervical spine.

Connections
Myofascial relationship and with the connective tissues associated with the articular disc of the wrist.

Brachioradialis

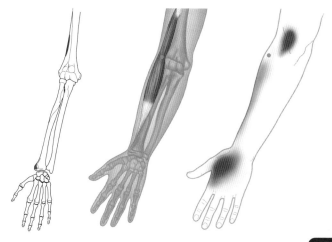

Latin, *brachium*, arm; *radius*, staff, spoke of wheel.

Brachioradialis forms the lateral border of the cubital fossa. The muscle belly is prominent when working against resistance.

Origin
Proximal part of lateral supraepicondylar ridge of humerus and adjacent intermuscular septum.

Insertion
Lower surface of distal end of radius, just above styloid process.

Nerve
Radial nerve C5, 6.

Action
Accessory flexor of elbow joint when forearm is midpronated.

Basic Functional Movement
Example: turning a corkscrew.

Referred Pain Patterns
Lateral epicondyle area 3–4 cm patch with vague arm pain (radius border), localizing into strong pain in dorsum of thumb.

Indications
Elbow pain, pain in thumb (dorsum), tennis elbow, weakness of grip, RSI.

Causes
RSI, prolonged mouse use, racquet sports, poor stretching, playing musical instruments.

Differential Diagnosis
De Quervain's tenosynovitis. Osteoarthritis of thumb (trapezium).

Connections
Biceps brachiii, brachialis, extensor carpi radialis longus/ brevis, supinator, extensor digitorum.

Wrist Extensors

Latin, *extendere*, to extend; *carpi*, of the wrist; *radius*, staff, spoke of wheel; *longus*, long; *brevis*, short; *ulnaris*, of the elbow.

Origin
Common extensor tendon from lateral epicondyle of humerus (i.e., lower lateral end of humerus).

Insertion
Dorsal surface of metacarpal bones.

Nerve
Extensor radialis longus/brevis: radial nerve, C5, 6, 7, 8.
Extensor carpi ulnaris: deep radial (posterior interosseous) nerve, C5, 6, 7, 8.

Action
Extends wrist joint (extensor carpi radialis longus/brevis also abduct wrist joint; extensor carpi ulnaris also adducts wrist joint).

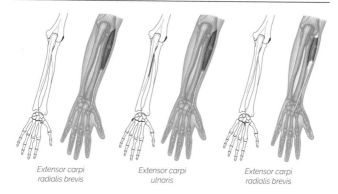

Extensor carpi radialis brevis

Extensor carpi ulnaris

Extensor carpi radialis brevis

Basic Functional Movement
Examples: kneading dough; typing; cleaning windows.

Referred Pain Patterns
Extensor carpi radialis longus: strong 2–3 cm zone over lateral epicondyle, diffusely radiating to dorsum of hand above thumb.
Extensor carpi radialis brevis: strong zone of pain 3–5 cm over dorsum of hand.

Extensor carpi ulnaris: strong, localized, specific referral to dorsal ulnar surface of hand and bulk of wrist.

Indications
Forearm/elbow/wrist/hand pain, finger stiffness, painful/weak grip, tennis elbow, pain on gripping and twisting, loss of control (fine) on gripping activities.

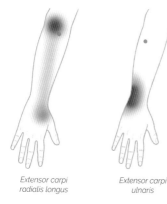
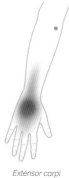

Extensor carpi radialis longus

Extensor carpi ulnaris

Extensor carpi radialis brevis

Causes

Computer mouse/keyboard, prolonged repetitive gripping (e.g., writing, ironing, using tools, throwing, massaging), wrist fractures or falls (extensor carpi ulnaris), casts, sports (e.g., racquet—tennis elbow, poles—skiing), occupational, playing musical instruments (piano, violin, drum).

Differential Diagnosis

Epicondylitis. C5–C6 radiculopathy. De Quervain's tenosynovitis. Articular dysfunction of wrist. Osteoarthritis. Carpal tunnel syndrome.

Connections

Supinator, brachioradialis, extensor digitorum, triceps brachii, biceps brachii, anconeus.

Extensor Digitorum

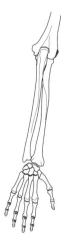 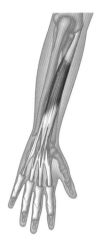

Latin, *extendere*, to extend; *digitorum*, of the fingers/toes.

Each tendon of extensor digitorum, over each metacarpophalangeal joint, forms a triangular membranous sheet called the *extensor hood* or *extensor expansion*, into which inserts the lumbricals and interossei of the hand. Extensor digiti minimi and extensor indicis also insert into the extensor hood.

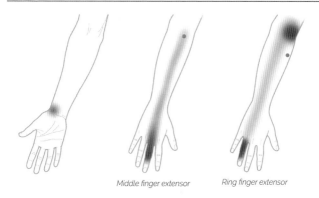

Middle finger extensor   *Ring finger extensor*

Origin
Lateral epicondyle of humerus and adjacent intermuscular septum and deep fascia.

Insertion
Four tendons, which insert via extensor hoods into the dorsal aspects of the bases of the middle and distal phalanges of the index, middle, ring, and little fingers.

Nerve
Posterior interosseous nerve C7, 8.

Action
Extends the index, middle, ring, and little fingers; can also extend the wrist.

Basic Functional Movement
Example: letting go of objects held in the hand.

Referred Pain Patterns
Diffuse pain from forearm, becoming more intense in the appropriate finger (proximal metacarpal). Pain in lateral epicondyle.

Indications
Finger/hand/wrist/elbow pain, stiffness/pain/weakness (decreased grip) in fingers, tennis elbow, pain on forceful gripping, often seen in professional musicians (esp. guitarists).

Causes
Computer mouse/keyboard, prolonged repetitive gripping (e.g., writing, ironing, using tools, throwing, massaging), wrist fractures or falls, casts, sports (e.g., racquet—tennis elbow, poles—skiing), occupational, playing musical instruments (e.g., piano, violin, drum), sleeping with hands curled under head/pillow.

Differential Diagnosis
Radiculopathy (cervical). Epicondylitis (tennis

elbow). Osteoarthritis of fingers. De Quervain's tenosynovitis. Mechanical wrist pain (carpals).

Connections
Brachioradialis, supinator, extensor carpi radialis longus, extensor indicis.

Supinator

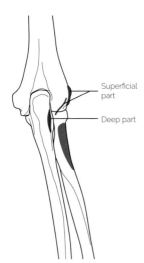
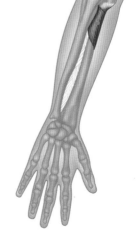

Superficial part

Deep part

Latin, *supinus*, lying on the back.

Supinator is almost entirely concealed by the superficial muscles.

Origin
Superficial part: lateral epicondyle of humerus. Radial collateral and anular ligaments.
Deep part: supinator crest of ulna.

Insertion
Lateral surface of radius superior to the anterior oblique line.

Nerve
Posterior interosseous nerve C5, 6, (7).

Action
Supination.

Basic Functional Movement
Example: turning a door handle or screwdriver.

Referred Pain Patterns
Localized 3–5 cm strong zone of pain at lateral epicondyle and at web of thumb (dorsum).

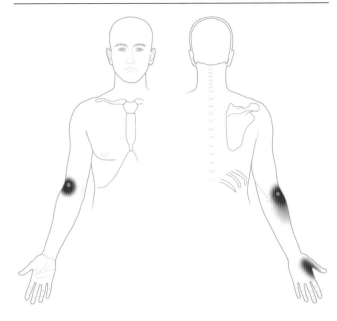

Indications
Tennis elbow, thumb joint pain, elbow pain (when carrying and at rest), pain turning doorknobs, localized pain on supination, chronic use of walking stick, pain on handshake.

Causes
Repetitive motions with straight arm (e.g., tennis, dog walking, carrying heavy case), repetitive motions (e.g., twisting, massaging, driving, ironing), trauma/strain, racquet sports.

Differential Diagnosis
De Quervain's tenosynovitis. Lateral epicondylitis (tendo-osseous, musculotendinous, intramuscular). Radial head dysfunction.

Connections
Common extensors, biceps brachii, triceps brachii (insertion), anconeus, brachialis, palmaris longus, brachioradialis, extensor carpi radialis longus.

Abductor Pollicis Longus

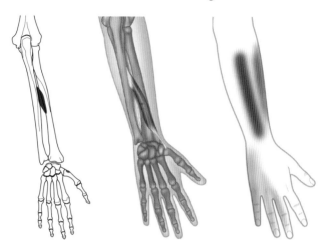

Latin, *abducere*, to lead away from; *pollicis*, of the thumb; *longus*, long.

Although part of the deep group of muscles, this muscle becomes superficial in the distal part of the forearm.

Origin
Posterior surfaces of ulna and radius, distal to attachments of supinator and anconeus. Intervening interosseous membrane.

Insertion
Lateral side of base of first metacarpal.

Nerve
Posterior interosseous nerve C7, 8.

Action
Abducts carpometacarpal joint of thumb; accessory extensor of thumb.

Basic Functional Movement
Example: releasing the grip on a flat object.

Referred Pain Patterns
The radial aspect of the wrist (61.9%), the dorsal aspects of the third and fourth fingers (14.3%), and/or a combination of the two pain patterns (23.8%).

Indications
Thenar region pain—thumb region pain aching and discomfort.

Causes
Occupational (massage) post fracture, O/A thumb, texter's thumb, overuse syndromes, mouse use, racquet sports, DIY, poor stretching, musical instruments (piano).

Differential Diagnosis
De Quervain's tenosynovitis, ulnar neuropathy, cervicogenic pain, and radiculopathy.

Connections
Abductor pollicis brevis.

Extensor Indicis

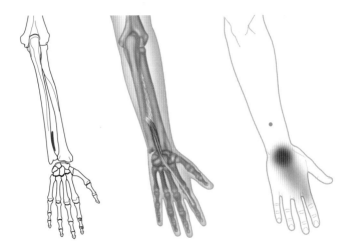

Latin, *extendere*, to extend; *indicis*, of the index finger.

Origin
Posterior surface of ulna, distal to extensor pollicis longus. Adjacent interosseous membrane.

Insertion
Extensor hood of index finger.

Nerve
Posterior interosseous nerve C7, 8.

Action
Extends index finger.

Basic Functional Movement
Example: pointing at something.

Referred Pain Patterns
Dorsal wrist and hand pain.

Indications
Pain located in the forearm and hand, finger stiff, painful, and may cause the finger to cramp.

Causes
Falls, mobile device overuse, RSI/occupational overuse, mouse, post-fracture splinting.

Differential Diagnosis
Wrist strain, fracture, Kienbock's disease, O/A.

Connections
Wrist extensors.

Opponens Pollicis and Adductor Pollicis

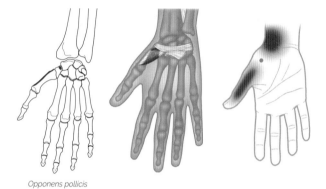

Opponens pollicis

Latin, *opponens*, opposing; *pollicis*, of the thumb.

Usually partly fused with flexor pollicis brevis and deep to abductor pollicis brevis.

Origin
Flexor retinaculum. Tubercle of trapezium.

Insertion
Entire length of radial border of first metacarpal.

Nerve
Recurrent branch of median nerve C8, T1.

Action
Medially rotates thumb.

Basic functional movement
Example: picking up a small object between the thumb and fingers.

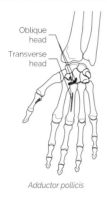

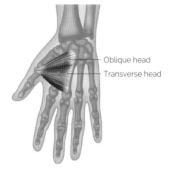

Adductor pollicis

Latin, *adducere*, to lead to; *pollicis*, of the thumb.

Origin
Transverse head: palmar surface of third metacarpal.
Oblique head: capitate and bases of second and third metacarpals.

Insertion
Base of proximal phalanx of thumb and extensor hood of thumb.

Nerve
Deep branch of ulnar nerve C8, T1.

Action
Adducts thumb.

Basic Functional Movement
Example: gripping a jam jar lid to screw it on.

Referred Pain Patterns
Opponens pollicis: palmar wrist pain at distal radial head and into palmar aspect of thumb.
Adductor pollicis: dorsal and palmar surfaces of thumb, localized around metacarpophalangeal joint and radiating to web of thumb and thenar eminence.

Indications
"Weeder's thumb," thumb pain on activity, difficulty maintaining pincer movement, "texter's/video gamer's thumb," pain sewing/writing/opening jars, loss of fine motor control (e.g., buttoning, sewing, writing, painting).

Causes
Post wrist/thumb fracture, wrist splinting, grasping with thumb, carrying shopping, texting, holding e-reader/tablet, massaging, fine handiwork (e.g., writing, sewing, knitting,

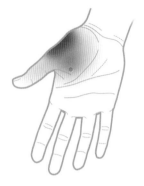
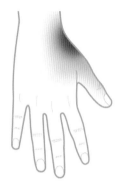

artwork, painting, airbrushing), playing musical instruments.

Differential Diagnosis
De Quervain's tenosynovitis. Osteoarthritis of thumb (saddle joint). Rheumatoid arthritis. Carpal tunnel syndrome. "Trigger thumb." Discopathy of distal radioulnar joint. Carpal bones dysfunction. Mechanical dysfunction. Fracture. Subluxation.

Connections
Abductor pollicis brevis, flexor pollicis brevis/longus.

Abductor Pollicis Brevis

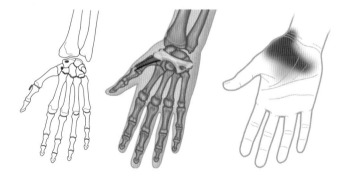

Latin, *abducere*, to lead away from; *pollicis*, of the thumb; *brevis*, short.

Origin
Tubercles of trapezium and scaphoid and adjacent flexor retinaculum.

Insertion
Proximal phalanx and extensor hood of thumb.

Nerve
Recurrent branch of median nerve C8, T1.

Action
Abducts thumb at metacarpophalangeal joint.

Basic Functional Movement
Example: typing.

Referred Pain Patterns
Localized to the region of the thenar eminence and thumb saddle joint.

Indications
Pain on gripping, aching in the thumb.

Causes
O/A of the thumb saddle joint. Trauma, prolonged gripping—cycling/driving. Occupational—esp. if there is a vibrational component (machines). Post-operative for replacing thumb joint, falling.

Differential Diagnosis
O/A of the thumb saddle joint. Carpal tunnel syndrome, carpal bone pathologies.

Connections
Opponens pollicis, abductor pollicis longus.

Small Hand Muscles

Latin, *dorsum*, back; *interosseus*, between bones; *lumbricus*, earthworm; *abducere*, to lead away from; *digitus*, finger; *minimi*, smallest.

The four dorsal interossei are about twice the size of the palmar interossei. The lumbricals are composed of small cylindrical muscles, one for each finger. The abductor digiti minimi is the most superficial muscle of the hypothenar eminence.

Origin
Dorsal interossei: by two heads, each from adjacent sides of metacarpals.
Lumbricals: tendons of flexor digitorum profundus in palm.
Abductor digiti minimi: pisiform bone. Tendon of flexor carpi ulnaris.

Insertion
Dorsal interossei: into extensor expansion and to base of proximal phalanx.

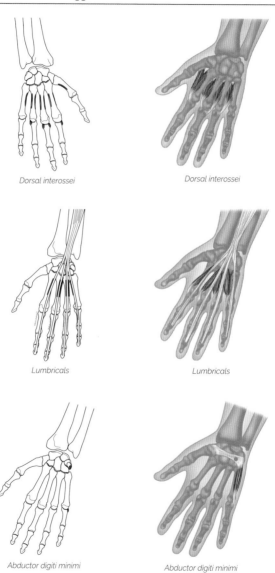

Dorsal interossei

Dorsal interossei

Lumbricals

Lumbricals

Abductor digiti minimi

Abductor digiti minimi

Lumbricals: lateral (radial) side of corresponding tendon of extensor digitorum, on dorsum of respective digits.
Abductor digiti minimi: ulna (medial) side of base of proximal phalanx of little finger.

Nerve
Dorsal interossei: ulnar nerve, C**8**, T**1**.
Lumbricals: lateral—median nerve, C(6), 7, **8**, T**1**; medial—ulnar nerve, C(7), **8**, T**1**.

Abductor digiti minimi: ulnar nerve, C(7), **8**, T**1**.

Action
Dorsal interossei: abduct fingers away from middle finger. Assist in flexion of fingers at metacarpophalangeal joints.
Lumbricals: extend interphalangeal joints and simultaneously flex metacarpophalangeal joints of fingers.
Abductor digiti minimi: abducts little finger.

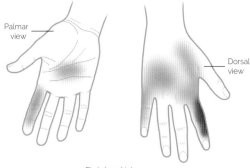

Palmar view

Dorsal view

First dorsal interosseous

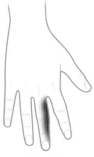

Dorsal view
Second dorsal interosseous

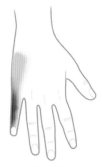

Dorsal view
Abductor digiti minimi

Basic Functional Movement

Examples: spreading fingers; cupping hand; holding a large ball.

Referred Pain Patterns

First dorsal interossei: strong finger pain in dorsum of index finger (lateral half), with vague pain on palmar surface and dorsum of hand. *Other dorsal interossei:* referred pain to specific associated finger.

Lumbricals: pattern is similar to interossei.

Abductor digiti minimi: pain in dorsum of little finger.

Indications

Finger pain/stiffness, pain when pinching/gripping, associated with Heberden's node(s) (e.g., in professional musicians, esp. pianists), "arthritic" finger pain, also seen in artists/sculptors, Bouchard's nodes (middle knuckles).

Causes

Repetitive grasping, occupational, computer mouse, post wrist fracture and/or splinting, grasping, carrying shopping, typing, massaging, fine handiwork (e.g., writing, sewing, knitting, artwork, painting, airbrushing), playing musical instruments (e.g., piano, violin, guitar), sports (e.g., golf, archery, fencing).

Differential Diagnosis

Cervical radiculopathy. Ulnar neuritis. Thoracic outlet syndrome. Digital nerve entrapment. Articular dysfunction.

Connections

Intrinsic thumb muscles, scalenes, latissimus dorsi, long finger flexors/extensors, pectoralis major, lateral/medial head triceps brachii (lateral/medial heads).

Trigger Points and Carpal Tunnel Syndrome

Carpal Tunnel Syndrome (CTS) is the single most common form of entrapment neuropathy. It involves pressure on the median nerve of the wrist beneath non-flexible structures at the wrist.

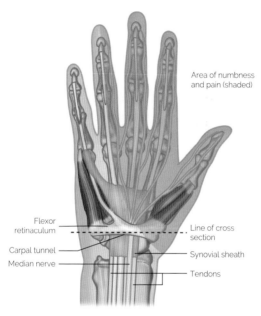

Area of numbness and pain (shaded)

Flexor retinaculum

Carpal tunnel

Median nerve

Line of cross section

Synovial sheath

Tendons

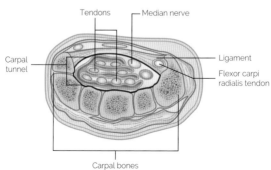

Tendons

Median nerve

Carpal tunnel

Ligament

Flexor carpi radialis tendon

Carpal bones

Sustained, high pressure in the tunnel impedes microcirculation in the median nerve leading eventually to decreased action potentials, demyelination in the nerve, and axonal degeneration. There may also be an entrapment from tight muscles, it is well worth looking at trigger points in the **pronator teres** (page 134) and **palmaris longus** (page 135) to relieve or even significantly improve the symptoms.

Numbness or tingling of the thumb and fingers—particularly the index and middle fingers—is one of the most common symptoms of CTS. This sensation is often felt when holding a steering wheel, phone, or newspaper. Weakness in the hands is also a common symptom of CTS, leading to a tendency to drop objects. Weakness usually develops after numbness or tingling.

Symptoms of CTS develop gradually but tend to worsen at night. This may be because of a sleep position, where wrists are flexed during sleep. Patients often feel the need to vigorously shake their wrists in the morning.

CHAPTER 6

Muscles of the Hip and Thigh

As low back pain has become increasingly common, so has hip pain, and it is no coincidence that many hip pain disorders occur as unnecessary secondary conditions to mismanaged low back pain disorders. Chronic trigger-point-induced muscle tension in the muscle groups that function to move the hip joint may even lead, over time, to hip joint damage. Three key hip-muscle trigger points referring pain to the hip joint are quadratus lumborum, tensor fasciae latae, and piriformis, although other muscles may be involved.

For tension in the muscles at the back of the thigh, consider trigger points in the hamstrings, gluteus minimus, and gastrocnemius. Posterior thigh pain is extremely common and may predispose to hamstring strains and tears in those who participate in athletics or other sports where heavy eccentric loads are involved. Trigger points in the hamstrings can refer pain to the buttocks, as well as to the back of the thigh/knee regions.

The normal functioning of the knee requires balance of muscular effort during walking, running, and other "knee loading" activities. Overload on the anterior thigh muscles can also refer pain to the knee joint, and beside the pain these trigger points may also cause a sudden buckling or weakness of the knee. Trigger points in the anterior thigh, including rectus femoris, vastus medialis, and vastus lateralis and sartorius, all can cause knee pain.

Gluteus Maximus

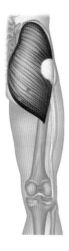 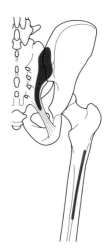

Greek, *gloutos*, buttock. *Latin*, *maximus*, biggest.

Gluteus maximus is the most coarsely fibered and heaviest muscle in the body. It is the strongest external rotator of the hip.

Origin
Fascia covering gluteus medius, external surface of ilium behind posterior gluteal line, fascia of erector spinae, dorsal surface of lower sacrum, lateral margin of coccyx, external surface of sacrotuberous ligament.

Insertion
Posterior aspect of ITB of fascia lata. Gluteal tuberosity of proximal femur.

Nerve
Inferior gluteal nerve L5, S1, 2.

Action
Powerful extensor of flexed femur at hip joint. Lateral stabilizer of hip and knee joints. Laterally rotates and abducts thigh.

Basic Functional Movement
Examples: walking upstairs, rising from sitting.

Referred Pain Patterns
Three to four strong zones of pain in buttock, with intercommunicating diffuse pain, occasionally just below (5–8 cm) gluteal fold.

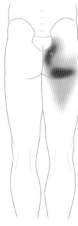

Middle superior

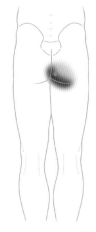

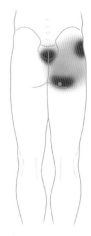

Middle inferior

Indications

Pain on sitting/climbing stairs/ walking (uphill), pain on flexion, buttock pain in cold water/when swimming/after a fall or trip, night pain, restricted hip/thigh flexion, listing gait, cramping in cold, pain in tailbone (coccyx zone), feels like "sitting on a nail" when on hard seat, low back pain, stiff hips.

Causes

Sitting on wallet in back pocket, prolonged occupational driving/ sitting (esp. when leaning back), sleeping on one side, swimming, trauma (e.g., fall), intramuscular injection, short leg (PSLE), spinal anomaly, sacroiliac joint dysfunction, climbing, certain office chairs/car seats.

Differential Diagnosis

Coccydynia. Pelvic inflammatory disease. Lower lumbar discopathy. Sacroiliitis. Bursitis (ischial tuberosity/trochanteric). Mechanical low back pain.

Connections

Other gluteal muscles, quadratus lumborum, pubococcygeus, hamstrings (attachment trigger points), abdominals.

Tensor Fasciae Latae

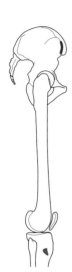 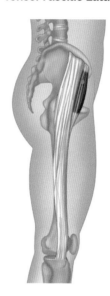 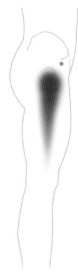

Latin, *tendere*, to stretch, pull; *fascia*, band; *lata*, side or lateral.

This muscle lies anterior to gluteus maximus, on the lateral side of the hip.

Origin
Lateral aspect of crest of ilium between ASIS and tubercle of the crest.

Insertion
Iliotibial tract which inserts into the upper lateral tibia.

Nerve
Superior gluteal nerve L4, 5, S1.

Action
Stabilizes the knee in extension.

Basic Functional Movement
Example: walking.

Referred Pain Patterns
Strong elliptical zone of pain from greater trochanter inferolaterally toward fibula.

Indications
Hip/knee pain (lateral), pain on side lying/fast walking/sitting with knees flexed up, hip-replacement rehabilitation, fracture of neck of femur rehabilitation, hip stiffness.

Causes
Foot pronation when running (compensating for foot problems), short leg, bursitis of hip, sacroiliac joint dysfunction, poor sit-up technique, climbing, lifting heavy loads, being overweight.

Differential Diagnosis
Trochanteric bursitis. Osteoarthritic hip. Sacroiliitis. Lumbar spondylosis.

Connections
Gluteals, vastus lateralis, rectus femoris, sartorius, quadratus lumborum, iliopsoas, paraspinals.

Gluteus Medius

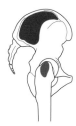 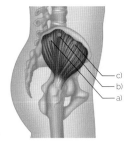

Greek, *gloutos*, buttock.
Latin, *medius*, middle.

Gluteus medius is mostly deep to, and therefore obscured by, gluteus maximus, but appears on the surface between gluteus maximus and TFL.

During walking, gluteus medius, along with gluteus minimus, prevents the pelvis from dropping toward the non-weight-bearing leg.

Origin
External surface of ilium between anterior and posterior gluteal lines.

Insertion
Oblique ridge on lateral surface of greater trochanter.

Nerve
Superior gluteal nerve L4, 5, S1.

Action

Abducts femur at hip joint. Medially rotates thigh. Holds pelvis secure over stance leg and prevents pelvic drop on the opposite swing side during walking (Trendelenburg gait).

Basic Functional Movement

Example: stepping sideways over an object, such as a low fence.

Referred Pain Patterns

Low back, medial buttock, and sacral and lateral hip, radiating somewhat into upper thigh.

Indications

Pain and tenderness in low back/buttocks (e.g., heavy lifting), night pain, pain on side lying, post hip or spinal surgery, sitting on wallet, leg length discrepancy, hip/back pain in bed, arthritic hip, hip pain, post hip fracture/surgery, pregnancy.

Causes

Sports injury (tennis, running, aerobics, upright biking), trauma from fall, motorcycling, injections in buttocks, standing on one leg, sitting cross-legged.

Differential Diagnosis

Radiculopathy (lumbosacral). Sacroiliitis. Hip joint dysfunction. Coccydynia. Greater tuberosity bursitis. Mechanical low back pain. Intermittent claudication.

Connections

Quadratus lumborum, other gluteal muscles, pubococcygeus, TFL, ITB, piriformis, lumbar erector spinae.

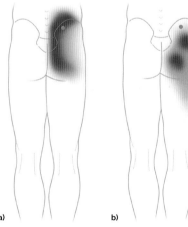
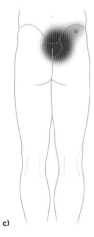

a)   b)   c)

Gluteus Minimus

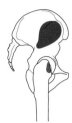 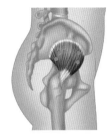

Greek, *gloutos*, buttock. **Latin**, *minimus*, smallest.

Gluteus minimus is situated anteroinferior and deep to gluteus medius, whose fibers obscure it. During walking, gluteus medius, along with gluteus minimus, prevents the pelvis from dropping toward the non-weight-bearing leg.

Origin
External surface of ilium between anterior and inferior gluteal lines.

Insertion
Anterolateral border of greater trochanter.

Nerve
Superior gluteal nerve L4, 5, S1.

Action
Abducts, medially rotates, and may assist in flexion of hip joint.

Basic Functional Movement
Example: stepping sideways over an object, such as a low fence.

Referred Pain Patterns
A multipennate muscle with multiple anterior, middle, and posterior trigger points referring strong pain in lower buttock, hip, and lateral lower extremity beyond knee to ankle and calf.

Indications
Pain sitting to standing, pain at rest/walking/side lying, night pain (may wake), hip replacement, sciatica/pseudosciatica, leg length discrepancy, postural issues, hip pain in bed, arthritic hip, post hip surgery.

Causes
Sitting on wallet, sports injury (tennis, running, biking), trauma from fall, motorcycling, standing on one leg, sitting cross-legged, hip/knee/ankle injury/fracture, leg casts.

Differential Diagnosis
Radiculopathy (lumbar). Sacroiliitis. Hip joint dysfunction. Sciatic irritation. Hip bursitis.

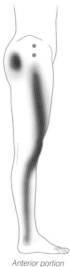
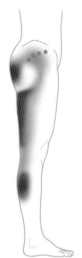

Anterior portion

Multiple trigger points

Connections
TFL, other gluteal muscles, vastus lateralis, ITB, quadratus lumborum, fibulares, piriformis, pelvic alignment.

Piriformis

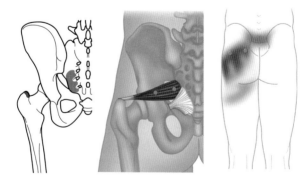

Latin, *pirum*, pear; *forma*, shape.

Piriformis leaves the pelvis by passing through the greater sciatic foramen, and along with obturator internus, is a muscle of the pelvic wall.

Origin
Anterior surface of sacrum between anterior sacral foramina.

Insertion
Medial side of superior border of greater trochanter.

Nerve
Branches from sacral nerves S1, 2.

Action
Laterally rotates extended femur at hip joint. Abducts flexed femur at hip joint. Helps hold head of femur in acetabulum. May assist with medial rotation when hip is flexed to 90 degrees and beyond.

Basic Functional Movement
Example: bringing the first leg out of a car.

Referred Pain Patterns
Two strong zones of pain:
(1) 3–4 cm zone lateral to coccyx;
(2) 7–10 cm zone posterolateral buttock/hip joint.
Also broad spillover of diffuse pain between (1) and (2) and down thigh to above the knee.

Indications
Constant "deep" ache in buttock, sciatica (pseudosciatica), vascular compression posterior legs, low back/buttock pain (worse when sitting), often starts after a fall or sitting on wallet when driving, foot/rectal/sacroiliac pain, sexual dysfunction (dyspareunia), piriformis syndrome (sciatica, local, and pelvic pain)—up to six times more common in women, pain worse on sitting.

Causes
Prolonged driving, trauma from fall, cycling/motorcycling, standing on one leg, hip surgery, sitting cross-legged, hip/knee/ankle injury/fracture, leg casts, high-heeled shoes, pelvic inflammatory disease (PID), sexual intercourse position, childbirth, arthritic hip, sacroiliac joint dysfunction, PSLE, improper/old orthotics.

Differential Diagnosis
Sacroiliitis. Lumbar radiculopathy. Coccydynia. Osteoarthritic hip. HLA (human leukocyte antigen)—B27 condition. Spinal stenosis. Discopathy (lumbar).

Connections
Leg length discrepancy, gluteal muscles, quadratus lumborum, attachment trigger point (origin) hamstrings, gemelli, obturators, quadratus femoris, levator ani, coccygeus.

"GIGO" Muscles

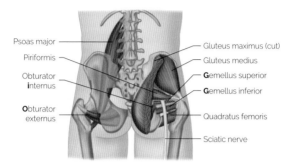

Psoas major
Piriformis
Obturator internus
Obturator externus

Gluteus maximus (cut)
Gluteus medius
Gemellus superior
Gemellus inferior
Quadratus femoris
Sciatic nerve

The short lateral rotators of the hip consist of (in anatomical sequence): gemellus superior, obturator internus, gemellus inferior, obturator externus, and quadratus femoris.

The muscles in this group often work together kinetically. They start at the top of the femur and run down, to insert on the posterior aspect of the femur and greater trochanter. Pain is generally felt locally—at the greater trochanter, over the buttock into the groin, and in the posterior thigh.

While it is often difficult to distinguish between the gemelli and the obturator muscles, the quadratus femoris is distal on the lower portion of the greater trochanter, which makes it somewhat more readily accessible. The gemelli and obturator muscles are difficult to treat with manual therapy but often respond well to dry needling. We will focus here on obturator internus.

Differential Diagnosis

Acute gluteal pain in athletes.
- Strains/avulsions
- Hamstring
- Gluteal
- Adductor
- External rotators
- Fracture
- Slipped capital femoral epiphysis
- Labral injuries
- Lumbar radiculopathies

Gemelli

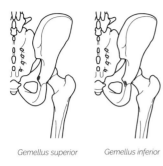

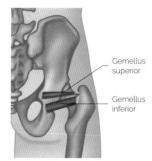

Gemellus superior

Gemellus inferior

Gemellus superior *Gemellus inferior*

Latin, *gemellus*, a twin/double; *superior*, upper; *inferior*, lower.

Origin
Superior: external surface of ischial spine.
Inferior: upper aspect of ischial tuberosity.

Insertion
Superior: along length of superior surface of obturator internus tendon and into medial side of greater trochanter with obturator internus tendon.
Inferior: along length of inferior surface of obturator internus tendon and into medial side of greater trochanter with obturator internus tendon.

Nerve
Superior: nerve to obturator internus, L5, S1.
Inferior: nerve to quadratus femoris, L5, S1, S(2).

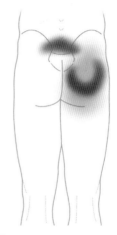

Action
Laterally rotate hip. Abduct flexed femur at hip joint. Help hold head of femur in acetabulum.

Basic Functional Movement
Example: bring first leg out of a car.

Referred Pain Patterns
Lumbopelvic pain, deep gluteal space pain, upper sacral/L5 area pain. Lancinating vaginal, rectal, scrotal, or posterior superior thigh pain.

Indications
Lumbopelvic pain, sitting buttock pain.

Causes
Hip-hitching, post-operative knee or hip, wearing a cast, using crutches, tight hip flexors (gemellus pain syndrome).

Differential Diagnosis
Posterior femoral cutaneous nerve entrapment syndrome, piriformis syndrome.

Connections
Piriformis, obturator internus, obturator externus.

Obturator Internus

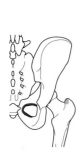 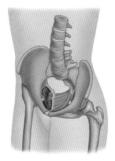 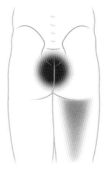

Latin, *obturare*, to obstruct; *internus*, internal.

Origin
Anterolateral wall of true pelvis; deep surface of obturator membrane and surrounding bone.

Insertion
Medial side of greater trochanter.

Nerve
Nerve to obturator internus, L5, S1.

Action
Laterally rotates hip joint. Abducts flexed femur at hip joint. Helps hold head of femur in acetabulum.

Basic Functional Movement
Example: bringing first leg out of a car.

Referred Pain Patterns
Local pain deep within pelvic basin and out as far as anterior medial portion of greater trochanter.

Indications
Pelvic pain, sitting buttock pain.

Causes
Hip-hitching, post knee or hip surgery, wearing a cast, using crutches, tight hip flexors (gemellus pain syndrome), postpartum damage.

Differential Diagnosis
Pudendal nerve entrapment. Posterior femoral cutaneous nerve entrapment syndrome. Piriformis syndrome.

Connections
Piriformis, gemelli.

Quadratus Femoris

Latin, *quadratus*, squared; *femoris*, of the thigh.

This small muscle helps to rotate the hip sideways. When the hip is flexed, it helps move the hip and thigh away from midline. The quadratus femoris is one of the short lateral rotator core muscles, which interact with dysfunctions of L4 through S3 vertebrae.

Movement is the best indicator as to which lateral rotator is involved. This muscle may stick to the underlying obturator externus. Patients who have active trigger points in the quadratus femoris will typically report pain, stiffness, and some difficulty walking, particular down hills or stairs. The pain from these TPs can be quite sharp, often sufficiently bad so that it interrupts sleep.

Some types of athletes are more prone than others to suffering from TPs in the quadratus femoris, esp. gymnasts and dancers.

Origin
Lateral edge of ischium just anterior to ischial tuberosity.

Insertion
Quadrate tubercle on intertrochanteric crest of proximal femur.

Nerve
Nerve to quadratus femoris, L5, S1, S(2).

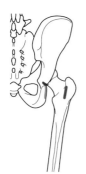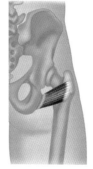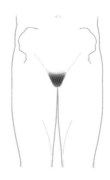

Action

Laterally rotates hip. Abducts flexed femur at hip joint. Helps hold head of femur in acetabulum.

Basic Functional Movement

Example: bringing first leg out of a car.

Referred Pain Patterns

Pain locally in posterior pubis and lower gluteal area. Difficulty in sleeping and walking downstairs are reported.

Trigger points in quadratus femoris typically appear locally together with other TPs in the immediate area, including the other short hip rotators, e.g., gemelli, and pelvic floor.

Sartorius

Latin, *sartor*, tailor.

Sartorius is the most superficial muscle of the anterior compartment of the thigh and is also the longest strap muscle in the body.

The medial border of the upper third of this muscle forms the lateral boundary of the **femoral triangle** (adductor longus forms the medial boundary, and the inguinal ligament forms the superior boundary).

The action of sartorius is to put the lower limbs in the seated cross-legged position of the tailor (hence its name from the Latin).

Origin

ASIS.

Insertion

Medial surface of tibia just inferomedial to tibial tuberosity.

Nerve

Femoral nerve L2, 3, (4).

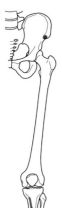 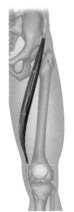 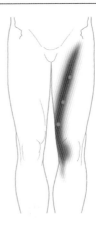

Action
Flexes the thigh at the hip joint (helping to bring leg forward in walking or running). Flexes the leg at the knee joint.

Basic Functional Movement
Example: sitting cross-legged.

Referred Pain Patterns
Vague tingling from ASIS anteromedially across thigh toward medial knee joint.

Indications
Ache in anterior thigh, sharp/tingling pain from hip to medial knee, pain after a twisting fall.

Causes
Gait/posture issues, sudden overload due to gymnastics, football/ice skating injury, horse riding, skiing, falling.

Differential Diagnosis
Meralgia paresthetica. Knee joint pathology. Lumbar radiculopathy. Inguinal lymphadenopathy. Vascular pathology. Inguinal and/or femoral hernia.

Connections
Vastus medialis, biceps femoris, gracilis, pectineus, TFL.

Quadriceps

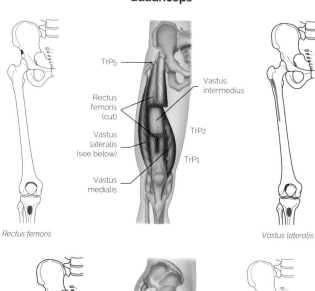

TrP5

Vastus intermedius

Rectus femoris (cut)

TrP2

Vastus lateralis (see below)

TrP1

Vastus medialis

Rectus femoris

Vastus lateralis

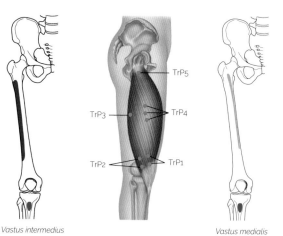

TrP5

TrP3

TrP4

TrP2

TrP1

Vastus intermedius

Vastus medialis

Latin, *rectus*, straight; *femoris*, of the thigh; *vastus*, vast; *lateralis*, relating to the side.

The four quadriceps (**Latin**: four-headed) femoris muscles all cross the knee joint, but the rectus femoris is the only that has two heads of origin: the reflected head is in the line of pull of the muscle in four-footed animals, whereas the straight head seems to have developed in humans as a result of the upright posture.

Vastus intermedius is the deepest part of the quadriceps femoris. This muscle has a membranous tendon on its anterior surface to allow a gliding movement between itself and the rectus femoris that overlies it.

The quadriceps femoris straighten the knee when rising from sitting, during walking and climbing. The vasti muscles as a group pay out to control the movement of sitting down.

Origin
Rectus femoris: straight head (anterior head): AIIS; reflected head (posterior head): groove above acetabulum (on ilium). *Vasti group:* upper half of shaft of femur.

Insertion
Patella, then via patellar ligament, into the tibial tuberosity.

Nerve
Femoral nerve L2, 3, 4.

Action
Rectus femoris: flexes the thigh at the hip joint (particularly in combination, as in kicking a ball), and extends leg at the knee joint. *Vasti group:* extend leg at the knee joint.

Basic Functional Movement
Examples: walking up stairs, cycling.

Referred Pain Patterns
Anterior, medial, and/or lateral thigh pain. Vastus lateralis has many points of pain referral.

Indications
Pain/weakness in thigh, "giving way" of knee, night pain, pain on knee extension, post hip fracture/femoral fracture and splinting, decreased femoropatellar joint "glide," pain on weight bearing, unexplained knee pain in young, pain/weakness descending stairs (rectus femoris), "toothache pain" near knee joint and "buckling" of knee (vastus medialis/intermedius), patellar tracking issues—chondromalacia patellae (vastus lateralis), jumper's/runner's knee, restless leg syndrome, meniscus pain.

Causes
Hamstring problems, sport/gym overloading or improper technique (esp. skiing, soccer, and squats), poor foot/ankle biomechanics, child/prolonged pressure on the lap.

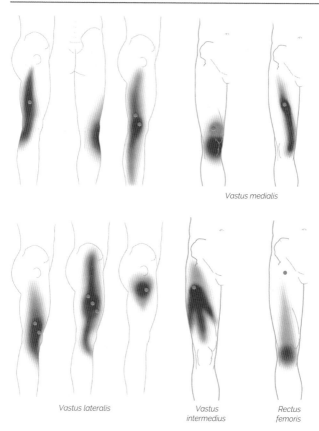

Vastus medialis

Vastus lateralis

Vastus intermedius

Rectus femoris

Differential Diagnosis

ITB syndrome, femoropatellar joint dysfunction, quadriceps expansion injury, tendinitis, lumbar radiculopathy, femoral nerve pathology, knee problems/dysfunction (multipennate).

Connections

Iliopsoas, TFL, gluteals, sartorius.

Gracilis

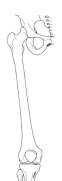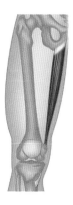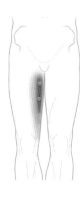

Latin, *gracilis*, slender, delicate.

Gracilis descends down the medial side of the thigh, anterior to semimembranosus.

There are five groin muscles used in adducting the hip, including the pectineus, adductor brevis, adductor longus, adductor magnus, and gracilis. Stretching the groin helps prevent strain injuries to the gracilis.

The gracilis is the most superficial of the adductors and lies in the midline of the medial thigh.

Origin
A line on the external surfaces of the pubis, the inferior pubic ramus, and ramus of the ischium.

Insertion
Medial surface of proximal shaft of tibia.

Nerve
Obturator nerve L2, 3.

Action
Adducts thigh at hip joint. Flexes leg at knee joint.

Basic Functional Movement
Example: sitting with the knees pressed together

Referred Pain Patterns
Medial thigh and anteromedial knee.

Indications
Linear pain in the medial thigh.

Causes
Horse riding, surfing, wakeboarding, certain exercise regimes.

Differential Diagnosis
Other adductor muscle, varicose veins.

Connections
Adductors.

Pectineus

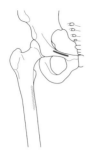 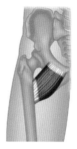 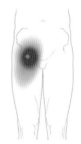

Latin, *pecten*, comb; *pectinatus*, comb shaped.

Pectineus is sandwiched between psoas major and adductor longus.

Origin
Pecten pubis and adjacent bone of pelvis.

Insertion
Oblique line, from base of lesser trochanter to linea aspera of femur.

Nerve
Femoral nerve L2, 3.

Action
Adducts and flexes thigh at hip joint.

Basic Functional Movement
Example: walking along a straight line

Referred Pain Patterns
Strong 8–12 cm zone of pain in anterior groin, with more diffuse radiations in an oval, toward the anteromedial thigh.

Indications
Persistent "internal" groin pain, groin strain, hip pain, post hip-replacement rehabilitation, post hip fracture, pregnancy, postpartum, pain during sexual intercourse/hip adduction exercises (gym), osteoarthritis of hip.

Causes
Leg splint/cast, foot/ankle problems, sudden overload due to gymnastics, football/ice skating injury, horse riding, skiing, cross-legged sitting.

Differential Diagnosis
Inguinal hernia. Femoral hernia. Lymphadenopathy. Meralgia paresthetica. Lumbar radiculopathy. Vascular incompetence.

Connections
Adductor longus/brevis, iliopsoas, leg length discrepancy.

Obturator Externus

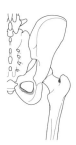 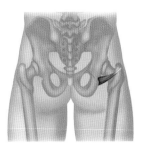 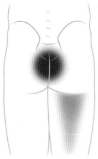

Latin, *obturare*, to obstruct; *externus*, external.

Origin
External surface of obturator membrane and adjacent bone.

Insertion
Trochanteric fossa.

Nerve
Posterior division of obturator nerve L3, 4.

Action
Laterally rotates thigh at hip joint.

Basic Functional Movement
Example: clicking the heels together "military style."

Referred Pain Pattern
Local pain deep within pelvic basin and out as far as posterior portion of greater trochanter.

If resisted, medial rotation causes increase in pain (sometimes pain shoots down medial aspect of femur).

Indications
Pelvic pain, sitting buttock pain.

Causes
Hip-hitching, post knee or hip surgery, wearing a cast, using crutches, tight hip flexors (gemellus pain syndrome), postpartum damage.

Differential Diagnosis
Pudendal nerve entrapment. Posterior femoral cutaneous nerve entrapment syndrome. Piriformis syndrome.

Connections
Piriformis, gemelli.

Adductors

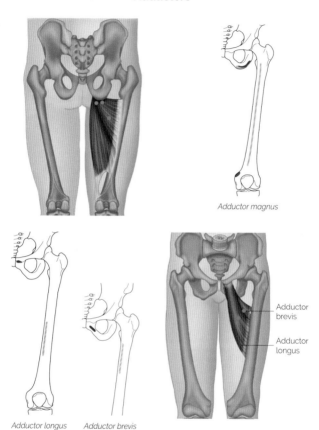

Adductor magnus

Adductor longus *Adductor brevis*

Adductor brevis

Adductor longus

Latin, *adducere,* to lead to; *magnus,* large; brevis, small; *longus,* long.

Adductor magnus is the largest of the adductor muscle group,

which also includes adductor brevis and adductor longus. Its upper fibers are often fused with those of quadratus femoris. Adductor longus is the most anterior of the three.

The lateral border of the upper fibers of adductor longus form the medial border of the **femoral triangle** (sartorius forms the lateral boundary; the inguinal ligament forms the superior boundary).

Origin
Anterior part of the pubic bone (ramus). Adductor magnus also takes its origin from the ischial tuberosity.

Insertion
Entire length of femur, along linea aspera and medial supracondylar line to adductor tubercle on medial epicondyle of femur.

Nerve
Magnus: obturator nerve L2, 3, 4. Sciatic nerve (tibial division) L2, 3, 4.
Brevis: obturator nerve L2, 3.
Longus: obturator nerve (anterior division) L2, 3, 4.

Action
Adduct and medially rotate thigh at hip joint.

Basic Functional Movement
Example: bringing the second leg in or out of a car.

Referred Pain Patterns
There are several zones of referred pain:

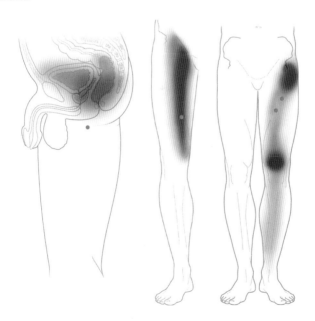

(1) two zones localized around anterior hip 5–8 cm, and above knee 5–8 cm;
(2) whole anteromedial thigh from inguinal ligament to medial knee joint;
(3) medial thigh from hip to knee.

Indications
Deep pain/tenderness in medial thigh, hip/leg stiffness on abduction, pain on weight bearing/rotating hip, "clicky" hip, hot/stinging pain under thigh, groin strain, post hip-replacement/fracture rehabilitation, renal tubular acidosis, swollen legs, osteoarthritis of hip.

Causes
Leg splint/cast, foot/ankle problems, sudden overload due to gymnastics, football/ice skating injury, horse riding, skiing, cross-legged sitting.

Differential Diagnosis
Avulsion. Pubic symphysis dysfunction. Neuropathy. Lymphadenopathy. Hernia. Knee pain (mechanical). Osteoarthritic hip. Femoral herniation.

Connections
Pectineus, vastus medialis, iliopsoas, vastus lateralis, sartorius (lower end).

Hamstrings

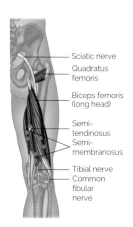

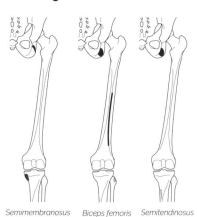

Semimembranosus   *Biceps femoris*   *Semitendinosus*

Latin, *semi*, half; *membranosus*, membranous; *tendinosus*, tendinous; *biceps*, two-headed; *femoris*, of the thigh.

The hamstrings consist of three muscles; from medial to lateral: semimembranosus, semitendinosus, and biceps femoris.

Origin
Ischial tuberosity. Biceps femoris (short head only): lateral lip of linea aspera.

Insertion
Semimembranosus: groove and adjacent bone on medial and posterior surface of medial tibial condyle.
Semitendinosus: medial surface of proximal tibia.
Biceps femoris: head of fibula.

Nerve
Sciatic nerve L5, S1, 2.

Action
Flexes leg at knee joint. Semimembranosus and semitendinosus extend thigh at hip joint, medially rotate thigh at hip joint and leg at knee joint. Biceps femoris extends and laterally rotates thigh at hip joint and laterally rotates leg at knee joint.

Basic Functional Movement
During running, the hamstrings slow down the leg at the end of its forward swing and prevent the trunk from flexing at the hip joint.

Referred Pain Patterns
Semimembranosus and semitendinosus: strong 10 cm zone of pain, inferior gluteal fold, with diffuse pain posteromedial legs to Achilles tendon area.
Biceps femoris: diffuse pain posteromedial legs, with strong 10 cm zone posterior to knee joint.

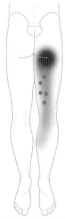

Semimembranosus/
Semitendinosus

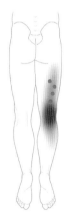

Biceps femoris
(short and long heads)

Indications

Posterior thigh pain sitting/
walking (worse at night),
tenderness in back of legs may
cause limping, pain worse
on sitting, post back surgery,
hamstring pain cycling/soccer/
basketball/tennis/football.

Causes

Prolonged driving, improper
sitting/work chair that digs
into back of thighs, hip surgery,
sitting cross-legged, hip/knee/
ankle injury/fracture, leg
casts, high-heeled shoes, PSLE,
sacroiliac joint dysfunction,
improper stretching before/after
sport.

Differential Diagnosis

Sciatica. Radiculopathy.
Muscle tears. Osteitis. Bursitic
osteoarthritis of knee. Knee joint
dysfunction. Tenosynovitis.

Connections

Piriformis, popliteus,
gluteals, obturator internus,
vastus lateralis, plantaris,
gastrocnemius, thoracolumbar
paraspinal muscles.

Trigger Points and Osteoarthritis of the Hip

Movements of the hip joint involve a particular pattern of sequential muscle activation. The specific patterns of muscular movement that we will look at are hip extension, hip abduction, as well as hip rotational movements. All of these patterns are made possible by the coordination of specific muscle groups. In general, the position for trigger points in the hip muscles will depend upon what the body is trying to achieve.

Hip Holding Patterns

Like a frozen shoulder (AC), osteoarthritis of the hip presents with a specific "default holding pattern" of flexion, adduction, and internal rotation. This leads to primary TPs in the (adduction): **Adductor magnus**, **adductor brevis**, and **adductor longus** (page 178), and secondary antagonist reciprocal inhibition in the **Gmed** (page 161) and **Gmin** (page 163). Also **psoas** (page 92) and **quadriceps femoris** (page 169) trigger points (flexion) and in the **pectineus** (page 176), **piriformis** (page 164), and short hip rotators (**"GIGO" complex**, page 166).

Similar to a frozen shoulder, this "hip holding" pattern is seen to a greater or lesser extent in most of the hip pain conditions (such as FAI).

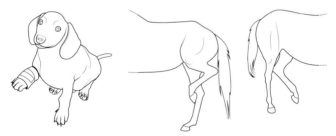

Hip holding patterns

Trigger Points and Buckling Knee

Knee buckling is relatively common among adults. In one study, adults aged 36–94 reported at least one episode of knee buckling in the past three months. It can affect people of all ages and levels of fitness.

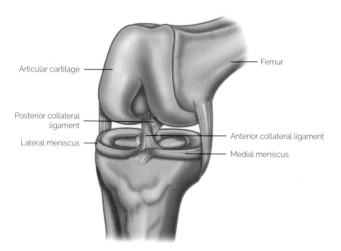

Articular cartilage

Femur

Posterior collateral ligament

Anterior collateral ligament

Lateral meniscus

Medial meniscus

This is an intriguing syndrome and is widely associated with TPs in the **vastus medialis** (page 172). It is often painless but sometimes painful, and manifests as a buckling of the knee in which the knee collapses. It has, at times, been mistaken for lumbar radiculopathy or also femoral plexus radiculopathy, but this is a misdiagnosis.

The diagnosis can be made by palpating the muscle and identifying TPs in the **vastus medialis**. Inactivating the TPs will immediately stop the knee from buckling. It is also worth looking at the antagonist muscles for TPs in long-standing or chronic conditions.

☑ Quadriceps—extension
☑ Hamstrings—flexion
☑ Stabilization—ITB from the Gmax and TFL

CHAPTER 7

Muscles of the Leg and Foot

Several conditions of the leg and foot can be associated with trigger points.

For plantar fasciitis, using good orthotics with arch supports may help. Consider trigger points in gastrocnemius, soleus, abductor hallucis, flexor digitorum brevis, abductor digiti minimi and/or quadratus plantae. Avoid running, jumping, prolonged driving > 40 minutes, and possibly walking until symptoms have subsided. Losing weight, if necessary, will help because extra weight puts additional stress on the leg and foot structures.

Hallux valgus is a painful condition where the big toe spreads out to the side at the joint closest to the foot, becoming deformed. Tightness and trigger points develop in flexor hallucis longus, and the bone can spread further owing to the forces exerted, making a self-perpetuating cycle. Flexor hallucis brevis, adductor hallucis, and abductor hallucis become weak, allowing even further spread and deformity. Patients should avoid wearing high heels.

Compartment syndromes, including shin splints (anterior compartment syndrome), are caused by swelling within the muscle compartment, leading to increased pressure, as a result of tight, short calf muscles. Symptoms include dull aching, tightness, and pain and develop over time, becoming worse after activity, with pain persisting for increased amounts of time after exercise.

For the *anterior* compartment, consider tibialis anterior, extensor hallucis longus, and extensor digitorum longus and brevis. For the *lateral* compartment, consider fibularis longus brevis and tertius. For the *superficial posterior* compartment, consider soleus and gastrocnemius; for the *deep posterior* compartment, flexor digitorum longus, flexor hallucis longus, popliteus, and tibialis posterior.

Tibialis Anterior

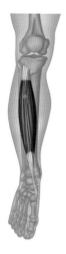 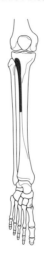 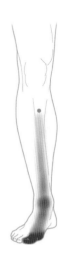

Latin, *tibialis*, relating to the shin; *anterior*, at the front.

Origin
Lateral surface of tibia and adjacent interosseous membrane.

Insertion
Medial and inferior surfaces of medial cuneiform and adjacent surfaces on base of first metatarsal.

Nerve
Deep fibular nerve L4, 5.

Action
Dorsiflexes foot at ankle joint. Inverts foot. Dynamic support of medial arch of foot.

Basic Functional Movement
Example: walking and running (helps prevent the foot from slapping onto the ground after the heel strikes, and lifts the foot clear of the ground as the leg swings forward).

Referred Pain Patterns
Anteromedial vague pain along shin, with zone of pain 3–5 cm in ankle joint (anterior), culminating in great-toe pain (whole toe).

Indications
Ankle pain/tenderness, pain in great toe, shin splints (anterior tibial compartment syndrome), foot dragging, ankle weakness (children), gout toe, turf toe, falls, balance issues.

Causes
Direct trauma, twisted ankle, ill-fitting boots/shoes, poor orthotics, walking on uneven surfaces, stubbing great toe, overload (e.g., walking, car pedals).

Differential Diagnosis
Lumbar discopathy. Arthritic toes. Anterior tibial compartment syndrome. Shin splints (anterior). Varicose veins.

Connections
Extensor hallucis longus, fibularis tertius, extensor hallucis brevis, extensor digitorum brevis/longus, flexor hallucis longus, first dorsal interosseous.

Extensor Digitorum Longus and Extensor Hallucis Longus

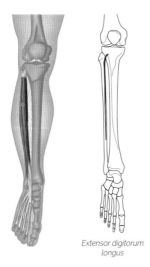

Extensor digitorum longus

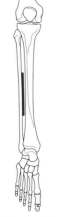
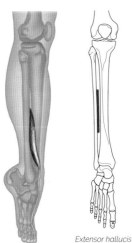

Extensor hallucis longus

Latin, *extendere*, to extend; *digitorum*, of the toes/fingers; *hallucis*, of the great toe; *longus*, long.

Like the corresponding tendons in the hand, extensor digitorum longus forms extensor hoods on the dorsum of the proximal phalanges of the foot. These hoods are joined by the tendons of the lumbricals and extensor digitorum brevis, but not by the interossei.

Origin
Extensor digitorum longus: proximal one-half of medial surface of fibula and related surface of lateral tibial condyle.
Extensor hallucis longus: middle one-half of medial surface of fibula and adjacent interosseous membrane.

Insertion
Extensor digitorum longus: along dorsal surface of the four lateral toes. Each tendon divides, to attach to bases of middle and distal phalanges.
Extensor hallucis longus: base of distal phalanx of great toe.

Nerve
Deep fibular nerve L5, S1.

Action
Extensor digitorum longus: extends lateral four toes and dorsiflexes foot.
Extensor hallucis longus: extends great toe. Dorsiflexes foot.

Basic Functional Movement
Example: walking up stairs (ensuring the great toe clears the steps).

Referred Pain Patterns
Extensor digitorum longus: pain in dorsum of foot, extending to middle three toes.
Extensor hallucis longus: pain over great-toe dorsum.

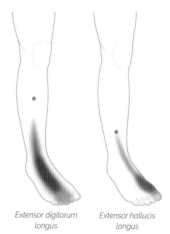

Extensor digitorum longus

Extensor hallucis longus

Indications
Dorsal foot pain, metatarsalgia, great-toe pain (pain is "persistent"), night cramps, anterior compartment syndrome, hammer/claw toe.

Causes
Direct trauma, twisted ankle, ill-fitting boots/shoes, poor orthotics, walking on uneven surfaces, stress fracture, splinting, stubbing great toe, sports (e.g., soccer, cycling, climbing).

Differential Diagnosis
Hammer/claw toes. Bunions. Lesions of fibular head. Compartment syndromes. Foot drop (upper motor neurone). Tendinitis. Tendon damage.

Connections
Fibulares, tibialis anterior.

Fibulares

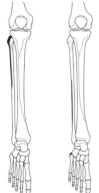
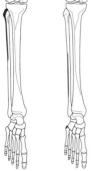
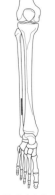

Fibularis longus   Fibularis brevis   Fibularis tertius

Latin, *fibula*, pin/buckle; *longus*, long; *brevis*, short; *tertius*, third.

The course of the tendon of the insertion of fibularis longus helps maintain the transverse and lateral longitudinal arches of the foot. A slip of muscle from fibularis brevis often joins the long extensor tendon of the little toe, whereupon it is known as *peroneus digiti minimi.*

Fibularis tertius is a partially separated, lower lateral part of extensor digitorum longus.

Origin
Fibularis longus: upper two-thirds of lateral surface of fibula, head of fibula, and occasionally lateral tibial condyle.

Fibularis brevis: lower two-thirds of lateral surface of shaft of fibula.
Fibularis tertius: distal part of medial surface of fibula.

Insertion
Fibularis longus: lateral side of distal end of medial cuneiform. Base of first metatarsal.
Fibularis brevis: lateral tubercle at base of fifth metatarsal.
Fibularis tertius: dorsomedial surface of base of fifth metatarsal.

Nerve
Fibularis brevis and longus: superficial fibular nerve L5, S1, 2.
Fibularis tertius: deep fibular nerve L5, S1.

Action
Fibularis longus: everts and plantar flexes foot. Supports arches of foot.
Fibularis brevis: everts foot.
Fibularis tertius: dorsiflexes and everts foot.

Basic Functional Movement
Example: walking on uneven ground; walking and running.

Referred Pain Patterns
Mainly over lateral malleolus, anteriorly and posteriorly in a linear distribution. Laterally along foot, occasionally vague pain in middle third of lateral aspect of lower leg.

Indications
Pronation of feet, repetitive inversion/eversion injury, tenderness around malleolus, ankle weakness, post-fracture (and casting) rehabilitation, foot problems (e.g., calluses, verrucae, neuromas), osteoarthritis of toes, metatarsalgia, ankle stiffness, lateral compartment syndrome.

Causes
Direct trauma, post-fracture, twisted ankle, ill-fitting boots/shoes, poor orthotics, walking on uneven surfaces, splinting (cast), sports (e.g., running, soccer,

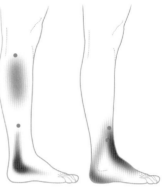

Fibularis longus (top), fibularis brevis (lower)

Fibularis tertius

cycling, climbing, swimming), footwear (high heels), tight socks, prolonged crossed legs, sleeping on stomach with pointed toes.

Differential Diagnosis
Rupture. Fracture of foot. Fracture of first metatarsal (styloid process). Foot problems. Fibular head dysfunction (common fibular nerve). Toe problems. Ankle problems (arthritis). Gait dysfunction. Compartment syndromes (lateral). Osteoarthritis of hip.

Connections
TFL, gluteus minimus, extensor digitorum longus/brevis, extensor hallucis brevis.

Gastrocnemius

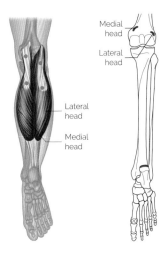

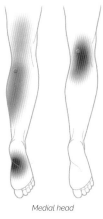

Medial head

Lateral head

Greek, *gaster*, stomach; *kneme*, lower leg.

Origin
Medial head: posterior surface of distal femur just superior to medial condyle.
Lateral head: upper postero-lateral surface of lateral femoral condyle.

Insertion
Posterior surface of calcaneus via the Achilles tendon.

Nerve
Tibial nerve S1, 2.

Action
Plantar flexes foot. Flexes knee. It is a main propelling force in walking and running.

Basic Functional Movement
Example: standing on tiptoes.

Referred Pain Patterns
Several trigger points in each muscle belly, and attachment trigger point at ankle. The four most common points are

indicated diagrammatically for medial and lateral heads.

Indications
Calf pain/stiffness, nocturnal cramps, foot pain (instep), pain in back of knee on mechanical activity, flat footed (dropped arches).

Causes
Direct trauma, post-fracture, twisted ankle, ill-fitting boots/shoes, poor orthotics, walking on uneven surfaces (uphill), splinting (cast), prolonged driving, occupational, (squatting) sports (e.g., running, soccer, cycling, climbing, swimming), footwear (high heels), tight socks, prolonged crossed legs, sleeping on stomach with pointed toes, calf cramps, biochemical (vitamin/mineral), drug-induced (side effects).

Differential Diagnosis
Thrombophlebitis. Deep vein thrombosis (varicose veins, intermittent claudication). S1 radiculopathy. Baker's cyst. Posterior tibial compartment syndrome. Achilles tendinitis. Sever's disease. Bursitis.

Connections
Soleus, plantaris, tibialis anterior/posterior, toe flexors (long), toe extensors.

Plantaris

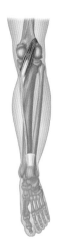 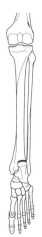 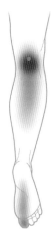

Latin, *plantaris*, relating to the sole.

Its long slender tendon is equivalent to the tendon of palmaris longus in the arm. Plantaris is absent in about 8–12% of the population, and is considered an unimportant muscle, acting mainly with gastrocnemius.

Origin
Lower part of lateral supracondylar line of femur and oblique popliteal ligament of knee joint.

Insertion
Posterior surface of calcaneus via the Achilles tendon.

Nerve
Tibial nerve S1, 2.

Action
Plantar flexes foot. Flexes knee.

Basic Functional Movement
Example: standing on tiptoes.

Referred Pain Patterns
Popliteal fossa pain in 2–3 cm zone, radiating 5–10 cm inferiorly into calf.

Indications
Calf/heel/posterior knee pain, chronic and long-term use of high-heeled shoes, flat footed (dropped arches), shin splints, pain ascending stairs, growing pains in children.

Causes
Post-fracture, poor orthotics, prolonged driving, sports (e.g., running, soccer, cycling, climbing, swimming), footwear (high heels), tight socks, sitting with leg resting on chair/table, PSLE.

Differential Diagnosis
Achilles tendinitis. Compartment syndrome. Vascular disease. Heel spur. Fasciitis. Subtalar joint problems. Venous pump mechanisms. Tendon rupture. Baker's cyst. Shin splints. Stress fracture. Leg length discrepancy.

Connections
Popliteus, gastrocnemius, tibialis posterior, quadratus plantae (of foot), abductor hallucis (of foot), gluteus minimus.

Soleus

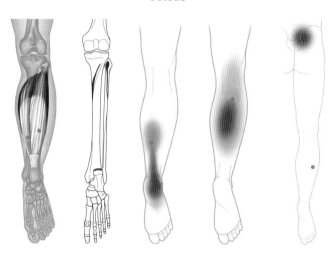

Latin, *solea*, leather sole/sandal/sole (fish).

Known as the skeletal muscle pump due to its responsibility for pumping venous blood back toward the heart from the periphery during upright posture.

Origin
Posterior aspect of fibular head and adjacent surfaces of neck and proximal shaft. Soleal line and medial border of tibia. Tendinous arch between tibial and fibular attachments.

Insertion
Posterior surface of calcaneus via the Achilles tendon.

Nerve
Tibial nerve S1, 2.

Action
Plantar flexes foot. Soleus is frequently in contraction during standing, to prevent the body falling forward at the ankle joint. Thus, it helps to maintain an upright posture.

Basic Functional Movement
Example: standing on tiptoes.

Referred Pain Patterns
Pain in distal Achilles tendon and heel to posterior half of foot. Calf pain from knee to just above Achilles tendon origin. 4–5 cm zone of pain in ipsilateral sacroiliac region (rare).

Indications

Calf/heel/posterior knee pain, chronic/long-term use of high-heeled shoes, plantar fasciitis, chronic calf shortening, calf pain walking stairs, low back pain, leg cramps.

Causes

Post-fracture splinting, poor orthotics, prolonged driving, sports (e.g., running, soccer, cycling, climbing, skiing, rowing machine), footwear (high heels), PSLE, occupational standing, direct blow/trauma, pressure on calf.

Differential Diagnosis

Achilles tendinitis. Compartment syndrome. Vascular disease. Heel spur. Fasciitis. Subtalar joint problems. Venous pump mechanisms. Tendon rupture. Baker's cyst. Shin splints. Stress fracture. Leg length discrepancy.

Connections

Popliteus, gastrocnemius, tibialis posterior, quadratus plantae (of foot), abductor hallucis (of foot), piriformis, occasionally to jaw.

Popliteus

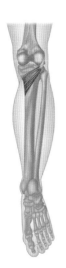
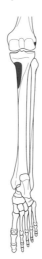
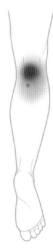

Latin, *poples*, knee, ham.

Origin
Lateral femoral condyle.

Insertion
Posterior surface of proximal tibia.

Nerve
Tibial nerve L4, 5, S1.

Action
Stabilizes and unlocks the knee joint.

Basic Functional Movement
Example: walking.

Referred Pain Patterns
Localized 5–6 cm zone of pain (posterior and central knee joint), with some spreading of diffuse pain, radiating in all directions, esp. inferiorly.

Indications
Pain in back of knee squatting/crouching/walking/running, pain behind knee/calf walking uphill and descending stairs, stiff knee on passive flexion/extension, plantar fasciitis, chronic calf shortening, low back pain, leg cramps.

Causes
Post-fracture, splinting, poor orthotics, prolonged driving, twisting sports (e.g., soccer, climbing, skiing, baseball, football), associated with many knee problems.

Differential Diagnosis
Avulsion. Cruciate ligaments (instability). Baker's cyst. Osteoarthritis. Tendinitis. Cartilage (meniscus) injury. Vascular (deep vein thrombosis, thrombosis). Tenosynovitis.

Connections
Biceps femoris, gastrocnemius (ligamentum patellae), plantaris.

Flexor Digitorum Longus and Flexor Hallucis Longus

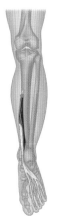
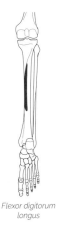

Flexor digitorum longus

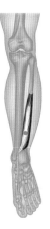
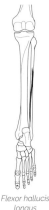

Flexor hallucis longus

Latin, *flectere*, to bend; *digitorum*, of the toes/fingers; *hallucis*, of the great toe; *longus*, long.

The insertion of the tendons of flexor digitorum longus into the lateral four toes parallels the insertion of flexor digitorum profundus in the hand.

Flexor hallucis longus helps maintain the medial longitudinal arch of the foot.

Origin
Flexor digitorum longus: medial side of posterior surface of tibia, below soleal line.
Flexor hallucis longus: lower two-thirds of posterior surface of fibula and adjacent interosseous membrane.

Insertion
Flexor digitorum longus: plantar surfaces of bases of distal phalanges of lateral four toes.
Flexor hallucis longus: plantar surface of base of distal phalanx of great toe.

Nerve
Tibial nerve S2, 3.

Action
Flexor digitorum longus: flexes lateral four toes (enabling the foot to firmly grip the ground when walking).
Flexor hallucis longus: flexes great toe, and is important in the final propulsive thrust of the foot during walking.

Basic Functional Movement

Examples: pushing off the surface in walking (esp. bare foot on uneven ground), standing on tiptoes.

Referred Pain Patterns

Flexor digitorum longus: vague linear pain in medial aspect of calf, with main symptoms of plantar forefoot pain.

Flexor hallucis longus: strong pain in great toe, both plantar and into first metatarsal head.

Indications

Foot pain on weight bearing/uneven surfaces, great-toe pain, leg cramps, numbness under great toe.

Causes

Arthritic (great) toes, poor footwear/orthotics, sports (e.g., walking, jogging, running), hypomobile ankles, flat feet, gout toe.

Differential Diagnosis

Shin splints. Compartment syndromes. Tendon ruptures.

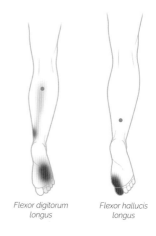

Flexor digitorum longus

Flexor hallucis longus

Instability of foot/ankle (medial). Stress (march) fracture. Morton's neuroma. Hammer toe/claw toe. Hallux valgus. Metatarsalgia. Osteoarthritis of first metatarsophalangeal joint. Gout. Plantar fasciitis.

Connections

Superficial/deep intrinsic foot muscles, tibialis posterior, long/short extensors of toes.

Tibialis Posterior

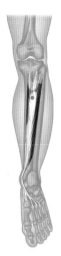 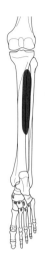 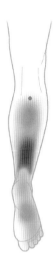

Latin, *tibialis*, relating to the shin; *posterior*, at the back.

Origin
Posterior surfaces of interosseous membrane and adjacent regions of tibia and fibula.

Insertion
Mainly to tuberosity of navicular and adjacent region of medial cuneiform.

Nerve
Tibial nerve L4, 5.

Action
Inverts and plantar flexes foot. Support of medial arch of the foot during walking.

Basic Functional Movement
Examples: standing on tiptoes, pushing down car pedals.

Referred Pain Patterns
Vague calf pain, with increased intensity along Achilles tendon to heel/sole of foot.

Indications
Achilles tendinitis, calf/heel pain, plantar fasciitis, pain running/walking on uneven surface, Morton's neuroma, foot numbness in patch around metatarsals, toe cramps, hammer/claw toe, tarsal tunnel syndrome.

Causes

Arthritic toes, poor footwear (heels) or orthotics, sports (e.g., walking, jogging, running, sprinting), hypomobile ankles, flat feet, prolonged driving (pedals).

Differential Diagnosis

Shin splints. Posterior tibial compartment syndrome (deep).

Tendon rupture. Tenosynovitis. Cardiovascular. Achilles tendinitis. Deep vein thrombosis.

Connections

Flexor digitorum longus, fibulares, flexor hallucis longus, foot mechanics.

Superficial Muscles of the Foot

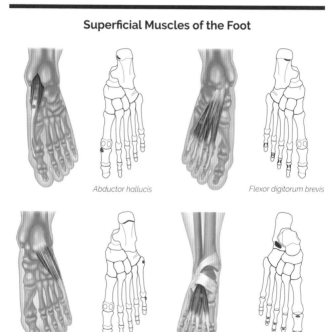

Abductor hallucis

Flexor digitorum brevis

Abductor digiti minimi

Extensor digitorum brevis

Latin, *abducere,* to lead away from; *hallux,* great toe; *flectere,* to bend; *digitus,* toe; *brevis,* short; *minimi,* smallest; *extendere,* to extend.

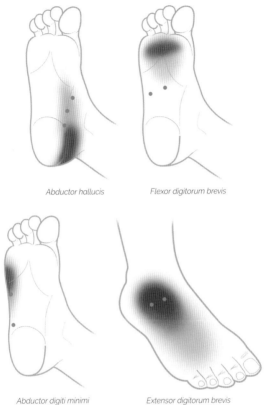

Abductor hallucis

Flexor digitorum brevis

Abductor digiti minimi

Extensor digitorum brevis

Comprising: abductor hallucis, flexor digitorum brevis, abductor digiti minimi, extensor digitorum brevis.

Origin
Abductor hallucis: tuberosity of calcaneus. Flexor retinaculum. Plantar aponeurosis.
Flexor digitorum brevis, abductor digiti minimi: tuberosity of calcaneus. Plantar aponeurosis. Adjacent intermuscular septa.

Extensor digitorum brevis: anterior part of superior and lateral surfaces of calcaneus. Lateral talocalcaneal ligament. Inferior extensor retinaculum.

Insertion
Abductor hallucis: medial side of base of proximal phalanx of great toe.
Flexor digitorum brevis: middle phalanges of second to fifth toes.

Abductor digiti minimi: lateral side of base of proximal phalanx of fifth toe.

Extensor digitorum brevis: base of proximal phalanx of great toe. Lateral sides of tendons of extensor digitorum longus to second to fourth toes.

Nerve

Abductor hallucis, flexor digitorum brevis: medial plantar nerve, L4, **5**, S1.

Abductor digiti minimi: lateral plantar nerve, S**2**, 3.

Extensor digitorum brevis: deep fibular nerve, L4, **5**, S1.

Action

Abductor hallucis: abducts and helps flex great toe at metatarsophalangeal joint.

Flexor digitorum brevis: flexes all joints of lateral four toes except distal interphalangeal joints.

Abductor digiti minimi: abducts fifth toe.

Extensor digitorum brevis: extends joints of medial four toes.

Basic Functional Movement

Examples: facilitating walking; helping foot stability and power in walking and running; helping to gather up material under foot by involving great toe.

Referred Pain Patterns

Abductor hallucis: medial heel pain, radiating along medial border of foot.

Flexor digitorum brevis: pain in plantar aspect of foot beneath (second to fourth) metatarsal heads.

Abductor digiti minimi: pain in plantar aspect of foot beneath fifth metatarsal head.

Extensor digitorum brevis: have a strong oval overlapping zone of pain (4–5 cm) in lateral dorsum of foot just below lateral malleolus.

Indications

Foot pain (dorsal/plantar), "soreness" on walking and "aching" at rest, pain on tiptoes/weight bearing/initial standing from sitting, chronic wear of high heels, Morton's neuroma, toe cramps, hammer/claw toe, patchy foot numbness.

Causes

Arthritic toes, poor footwear (heels) or orthotics, sports (e.g., swimming, walking, jogging, running, sprinting), hypomobile ankles, toe clawing, trauma.

Differential Diagnosis

Avulsion fracture of styloid process. Hallux valgus. Flat footed. Hallux rigidus or hypermobility. Metatarsalgia. Hammer/claw toe deformity. Heel spur. Stress (march) fracture. Compartment syndromes. Varus and valgus of foot.

Connections

Plantar interossei, quadratus plantae, adductor hallucis, extensor digitorum longus/brevis, flexor digitorum brevis, hip/knee/ankle/foot mechanics, extensor hallucis brevis, abductor hallucis.

Deep Muscles of the Foot

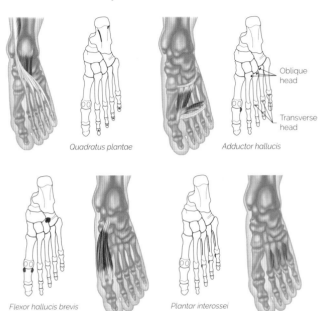

Quadratus plantae

Adductor hallucis

Oblique head

Transverse head

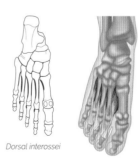

Flexor hallucis brevis

Plantar interossei

Dorsal interossei

Latin, *quadratus*, squared; *planta*, sole of the foot; *adducere*, to lead toward; *hallux*, great toe; *flectere*, to bend; *brevis*, short; *dorsum*, back; *interosseus*, between bones.

Comprising: quadratus plantae, adductor hallucis, flexor hallucis brevis, dorsal interossei, plantar interossei.

Origin
Quadratus plantae: medial head—medial surface of calcaneus; lateral head—lateral border of inferior surface of calcaneus.
Adductor hallucis: oblique head—bases of second to fourth metatarsals. Sheath of fibularis longus tendon; transverse head—plantar metatarsophalangeal ligaments of third to fifth toes. Transverse metatarsal ligaments.

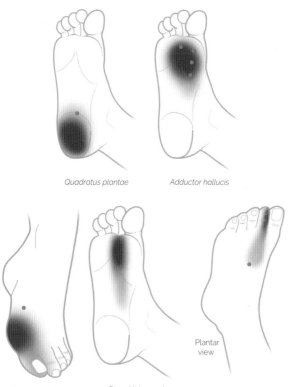

Quadratus plantae   Adductor hallucis

Plantar
view

Flexor hallucis brevis   Dorsal interossei

Flexor hallucis brevis: medial part of plantar surface of cuboid bone. Adjacent part of lateral cuneiform bone. Tendon of tibialis posterior.
Dorsal interossei: adjacent sides of metatarsal bones.
Plantar interossei: bases and medial sides of third to fifth metatarsals.

Insertion
Quadratus plantae: lateral border of tendon of flexor digitorum longus.
Adductor hallucis: lateral side of base of proximal phalanx of great toe.
Flexor hallucis brevis: medial part—medial side of base of proximal phalanx of great toe; lateral part—lateral side of base of proximal phalanx of great toe.

Dorsal interossei: bases of proximal phalanges: first—medial side of proximal phalanx of second toe; second to fourth—lateral sides of proximal phalanges of second to fourth toes.
Plantar interossei: medial sides of bases of proximal phalanges of same toes.

Nerve
Quadratus plantae, adductor hallucis, dorsal interossei, plantar interossei: lateral plantar nerve, S**1**, **2**.
Flexor hallucis brevis: medial plantar nerve, L4, **5**, S1.

Action
Quadratus plantae: flexes distal phalanges of second to fifth toes. Modifies oblique line of pull of flexor digitorum longus tendons to bring it in line with long axis of foot.
Adductor hallucis: adducts and assists in flexing metatarsophalangeal joint of great toe.
Flexor hallucis brevis: flexes metatarsophalangeal joint of great toe.
Dorsal interossei: abduct (spread) toes. Flex metatarsophalangeal joints.
Plantar interossei: adduct (close together) toes. Flex metatarsophalangeal joints.

Basic Functional Movement
Examples: holding a pencil between toes and ball of foot; helping to gather up material under foot by involving great toe; making a space between great toe and adjacent toe; facilitating walking.

Referred Pain Patterns
Quadratus plantae—heel pain; adductor hallucis—forefoot pain; flexor hallucis brevis—pain around first metatarsophalangeal joint; dorsal/plantar interossei—second digit pain (anteroposterior).

Indications
Foot/heel pain, pain in first metatarsophalangeal joint, bunions/hallux valgus, pain in 2nd toe, forefoot pain, stiffness in tissues (inability to use orthotic support), problems with walking, numbness in foot, hip/knee/ankle pain, heel spur, plantar fasciitis (quadratus plantae).

Causes
Arthritic toes, poor footwear (heels) or orthotics, sports (e.g., swimming, walking, jogging, running, sprinting), hypomobile ankles, toe clawing, trauma, chilling in wet socks/cold water.

Differential Diagnosis
Morton's neuroma. Metatarsalgia. Plantar fasciitis. Heel spur. Stress fracture. Articular (joint) dysfunctions. Injured sesamoid bones. Lumbar radiculopathy (foot drop). Hallux valgus. Calcaneal compartment syndrome. Gout. Arthritis.

Connections
Hip/knee/ankle problems, flexor digitorum brevis.

Trigger Points and Heel Pain

Heel pain presents commonly in clinical practice and plantar fasciitis (PF) is the most common disorder which causes heel pain, making up for 11–15% of foot care complaints affecting adults.

The plantar fascia is a thick band of tissue that connects the calcaneus to the toes supporting the arch of the foot—when strained, it becomes weak, swollen, and inflamed.

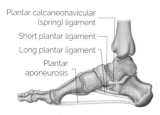

Plantar calcaneonavicular (spring) ligament
Short plantar ligament
Long plantar ligament
Plantar aponeurosis

Plantar fascia

Repetitive strain can bring about microtears in the soft tissues, leading to pain, swelling, and pre-disposing to further symptoms. Plantar fasciitis can be unilateral or bilateral.

Symptoms
Sharp pain that occurs with the very first steps in the morning. Once the foot "warms up," the pain of plantar fasciitis starts to decrease, appearing again after long periods of standing or from sitting to standing. Sudden stretching of the sole of the foot may increase the pain. In extreme cases, symptoms include numbness.

Fact Sheet
- Approximately 10% of people experience plantar fasciitis at some point in their lives.
- Plantar fasciitis most commonly arises in middle aged, obese females, and young male athletes.
- It may also occur in younger individuals who are on their feet for many hours of the day.
- It is particularly typical in runners and may occur if one starts running on a different surface, such as road instead of track.
- It may be associated with extreme pronation (inward rolling) of the foot, affected by flat feet.

Treating Heel Pain
In general, the main muscles to focus on for heel pain are **gastrocnemius** (page 191), **soleus** (page 194), **flexor digitorum longus** (page 197), and **tibialis posterior** (page 199).

For heel spur, the focus is on the **quadratus plantae** (page 203) muscle.

Advice—Never go barefoot while in recovery.

Dermatomes and Sensory Nerve Supply

Sensation from the skin is transferred to the spinal cord and hence to the brain by afferent nerve fibers which are part of the mixed, motor, and sensory nerves that make up the somatic peripheral nervous system.

All somatic nerves arise from one or more spinal segments and supply specific areas of skin. An area supplied by a single spinal segment is called a dermatome but the nerves supplying a single dermatome may be carried in one or more individual nerves.

A good example of this is the C5 dermatome in the upper limb, which is supplied by the C5 fibers carried in both the upper lateral cutaneous nerve of the arm (axillary nerve) and the C5 fibers in the lower lateral cutaneous nerve of arm (radial nerve).

The dermatomes and the distribution of the individual nerves images that follow have been compiled by the publisher with the guidance and assistance of Dr Robert Whitaker, MA, MD, MChir, FRCS, FMAA, Anatomist, University of Cambridge.

Cutaneous Nerves of the Arm

Anterior

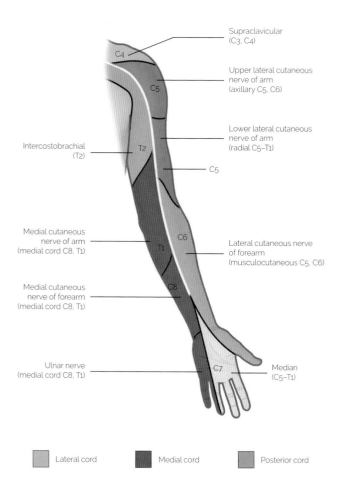

Supraclavicular
(C3, C4)

Upper lateral cutaneous
nerve of arm
(axillary C5, C6)

Lower lateral cutaneous
nerve of arm
(radial C5–T1)

C5

Intercostobrachial
(T2)

Medial cutaneous
nerve of arm
(medial cord C8, T1)

Lateral cutaneous nerve
of forearm
(musculocutaneous C5, C6)

Medial cutaneous
nerve of forearm
(medial cord C8, T1)

Ulnar nerve
(medial cord C8, T1)

Median
(C5–T1)

C4

C5

T2

C6

T1

C8

C7

☐ Lateral cord   ☐ Medial cord   ☐ Posterior cord

Posterior

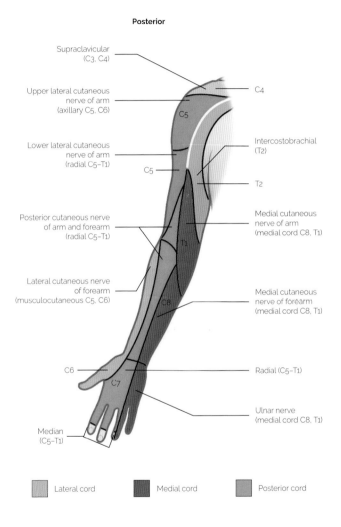

Supraclavicular
(C3, C4)

C4

Upper lateral cutaneous
nerve of arm
(axillary C5, C6)

C5

Lower lateral cutaneous
nerve of arm
(radial C5–T1)

C5

Intercostobrachial
(T2)

T2

Posterior cutaneous nerve
of arm and forearm
(radial C5–T1)

T1

Medial cutaneous
nerve of arm
(medial cord C8, T1)

Lateral cutaneous nerve
of forearm
(musculocutaneous C5, C6)

C8

Medial cutaneous
nerve of forearm
(medial cord C8, T1)

C6

C7

Radial (C5–T1)

Ulnar nerve
(medial cord C8, T1)

Median
(C5–T1)

Lateral cord

Medial cord

Posterior cord

Cutaneous Nerves of the Leg

Anterior

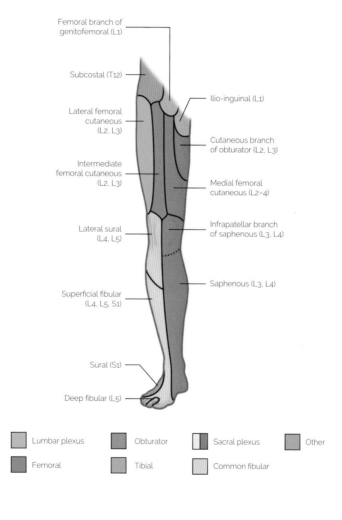

Femoral branch of genitofemoral (L1)

Subcostal (T12)

Lateral femoral cutaneous (L2, L3)

Intermediate femoral cutaneous (L2, L3)

Lateral sural (L4, L5)

Superficial fibular (L4, L5, S1)

Sural (S1)

Deep fibular (L5)

Ilio-inguinal (L1)

Cutaneous branch of obturator (L2, L3)

Medial femoral cutaneous (L2–4)

Infrapatellar branch of saphenous (L3, L4)

Saphenous (L3, L4)

Lumbar plexus

Femoral

Obturator

Tibial

Sacral plexus

Common fibular

Other

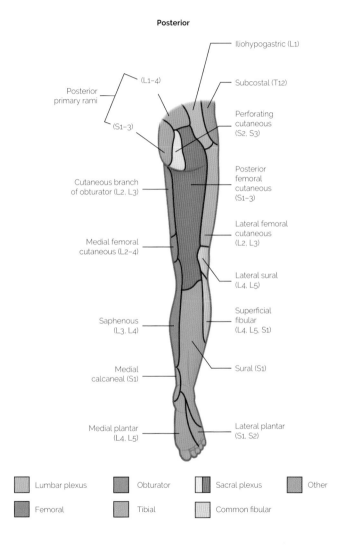

Posterior

Iliohypogastric (L1)

(L1–4)

Subcostal (T12)

Posterior primary rami

Perforating cutaneous (S2, S3)

(S1–3)

Posterior femoral cutaneous (S1–3)

Cutaneous branch of obturator (L2, L3)

Lateral femoral cutaneous (L2, L3)

Medial femoral cutaneous (L2–4)

Lateral sural (L4, L5)

Superficial fibular (L4, L5, S1)

Saphenous (L3, L4)

Medial calcaneal (S1)

Sural (S1)

Medial plantar (L4, L5)

Lateral plantar (S1, S2)

Lumbar plexus	Obturator	Sacral plexus	Other
Femoral	Tibial	Common fibular	

Anterior and Posterior Dermatomes

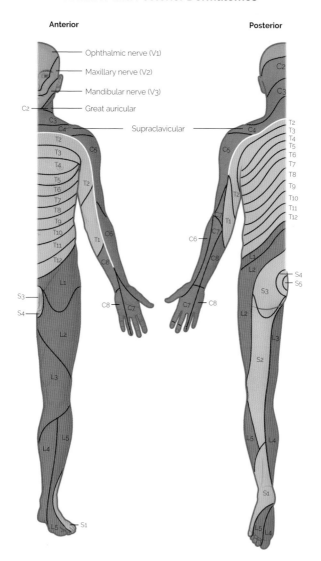

Anterior

Posterior

Ophthalmic nerve (V1)

Maxillary nerve (V2)

Mandibular nerve (V3)

Great auricular

Supraclavicular

Super Trigger Points

In the author's opinion, releasing trigger points in these muscles appears to have greater systemic effects than expected, often including profound physiological effects. Incorporating these "super trigger points" into a treatment protocol acts as a "shortcut," rapidly releasing deep-seated and chronic pain syndromes.

Anterior Super Trigger Points

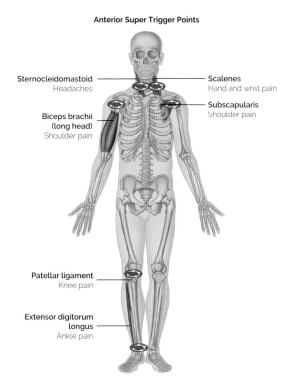

Sternocleidomastoid
Headaches

Scalenes
Hand and wrist pain

Subscapularis
Shoulder pain

Biceps brachii
(long head)
Shoulder pain

Patellar ligament
Knee pain

Extensor digitorum
longus
Ankle pain

Posterior Super Trigger Points

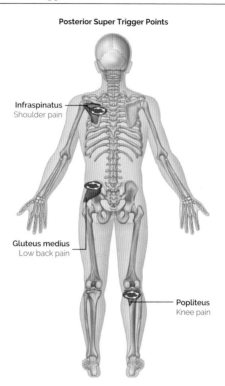

Infraspinatus
Shoulder pain

Gluteus medius
Low back pain

Popliteus
Knee pain

References

Davies, C. 2004. *The Trigger Point Therapy Workbook, Second Edition*. New Harbinger: Oakland.

DeLaune, V. 2011. *Pain Relief with Trigger Point Self-Help*. Lotus Publishing: Chichester.

Dommerholt, J., Bron, C., & Franssen, J. 2006. Myofascial Trigger Points: An Evidence-Informed Review. *J Man Manip Ther* **14**(4):203–221.

Drake, R., Wayne Vogel, A. & Mitchell, M. 2019. *Gray's Anatomy for Students, Fourth Edition*. Elsevier: London.

Gerwin, R.D., Dommerholt, J. & Shah, J.P. 2004. An Expansion of Simons' Integrated Hypothesis of Trigger Point Formation. *Curr Pain Headache Rep* **8**:468–475.

Hacket, G.S. 1991. *Ligament and Tendon Relaxation Treated by Prolotherapy, Third Edition*. Institute in Basic Life Principles.

Janda, V. 2005. Muscle Weakness and Inhibition in Back Pain Syndromes. In: Boyling, J.D., & Jull, G.A., *Grieve's Modern Manual Therapy: The Vertebral Column, Third Edition*, 197–201. Churchill Livingstone: Edinburgh.

Jarmey, C. 2018. *The Concise Book of Muscles, Fourth Edition*. Lotus Publishing: Chichester.

Jarmey, C. 2022. *The Pocket Atlas of Human Anatomy, Revised Edition*. Lotus Publishing: Chichester.

Lewit, K. 1999. *Manipulative Therapy in Rehabilitation of the Locomotor System, Third Edition*. Butterworth Heineman: London.

Myers, T. & Earls, J. 2017. *Fascial Release for Structural Balance, Revised Edition*. Lotus Publishing: Chichester.

Myers, T. 2020. *Anatomy Trains: Myofascial Meridians for Manual and Movement Therapists, Fourth Edition*. Elsevier: London.

Niel-Asher, S. 2014. *The Concise Book of Trigger Points: A Professional and Self-Help Manual, Third Edition*. Lotus Publishing: Chichester.

Schleip, R. 2020. *Fascial Fitness, Second Edition*. Lotus Publishing: Chichester.

Simons, D.G., Travell, J.G., & Simons, L.S. 1998. *Travell and Simons' Myofascial Pain and Dysfunction*, Vol. 1, Second Edition. Lippincott Williams & Wilkins: Baltimore, MD.

Starlanyl, D., & Sharkey, J. 2013. *Healing through Trigger Point Therapy*. Lotus Publishing: Chichester.

Travell, J.G., & Simons, D.G. 1992. *Myofascial Pain and Dysfunction*, Vol. 2. Lippincott Williams & Wilkins: Baltimore, MD.

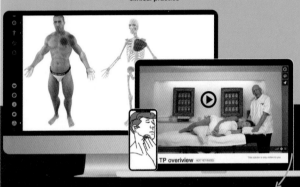